# Optimizing Brain Fitness

## Richard Restak, M.D.

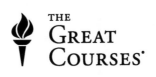

THE
GREAT
COURSES

PUBLISHED BY:

**THE GREAT COURSES**
**Corporate Headquarters**
**4840 Westfields Boulevard, Suite 500**
**Chantilly, Virginia 20151-2299**
**Phone: 1-800-832-2412**
**Fax: 703-378-3819**
**www.thegreatcourses.com**

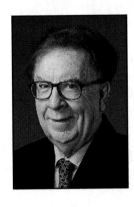

# Richard Restak, M.D.

Clinical Professor of Neurology
The George Washington University School
of Medicine and Health Sciences

P rofessor Richard Restak is Clinical Professor of Neurology at The George Washington University School of Medicine and Health Sciences. He also maintains an active private practice in neurology and neuropsychiatry in Washington DC.

A graduate of Georgetown University School of Medicine, Dr. Restak completed his postgraduate training at St. Vincent's Hospital in New York City, psychiatric training at Georgetown University Hospital, and a residency in neurology at The George Washington University Hospital.

Dr. Restak has written 20 books on the human brain, 2 of which were bestsellers and 4 of which were chosen as Main Selections of the Book-of-the-Month Club. He has penned dozens of articles for national newspapers, including *The Washington Post*, *The New York Times*, *Los Angeles Times*, and *USA Today*. He has contributed brain- and neuroscience-related entries for *World Book Encyclopedia*, *Compton's Encyclopedia*, *Encyclopedia Britannica*, and *Encyclopedia of Neuroscience*.

Dr. Restak has been elected to fellowship in the American Psychiatric Association, the American Academy of Neurology, and the American Neuropsychiatric Association. He served as president of the American Neuropsychiatric Association from 2005 to 2007. In 1992, the Chicago Neurosurgical Center awarded him the Decade of the Brain Award. In 1995, he received the Linacre Medal conferred by Georgetown University Medical School.

Dr. Restak's consulting appointments have included the Weill Music Institute at Carnegie Hall; the Franklin Institute Science Museum of Philadelphia;

the the Office of Interdisciplinary Studies, Smithsonian Institution; and the Advisory Panel, U.S. Congress Office of Technology Assessment. He has served on the Board of Advisors for the School of Philosophy at The Catholic University of America and was a member of the Board of Trustees at the Krasnow Institute for Advanced Study at George Mason University.

Dr. Restak has lectured regularly at the Smithsonian Associates. He has also delivered lectures at the Rubin Museum of Art in New York City; the Massachusetts Institute of Technology; the National Academies; the Library of Congress; the Brookings Institute; the 92nd Street Y in New York City; the National Security Agency; the Center for International and Security Studies at the University of Maryland School of Public Policy; the Johns Hopkins University Applied Physics Laboratory; the New York Academy of Sciences; the Philosophical Society of Washington; the FBI Academy; the Chautauqua Institute; the Franklin Institute Science Museum of Philadelphia; The Cooper Union; the National War College; the NASA Goddard Space Flight Center; the Society of Statesmen; the National Cryptologic School at the National Security Agency; and the Central Intelligence Agency.

Along with national and international lectures, Dr. Restak has presented commentaries for *Morning Edition* and *All Things Considered* on National Public Radio and has appeared on the *TODAY* show, *Good Morning America*, the Discovery Channel, and the *PBS NewsHour*. ■

# Table of Contents

# Table of Contents

# Optimizing Brain Fitness

**Scope:**

You can increase the power of your brain through your own effort. The brain's ability to change in response to experience—called plasticity—is the key to understanding the brain's development. The good news is that no matter how old you are, you can still take an active part in influencing brain plasticity. The brain is dependent on your experiences and continues to evolve throughout your lifespan.

In order to improve your brain, it's necessary to understand how it works. In this course you will learn how the brain is organized, how it develops, and how messages are transmitted through the brain's electrochemical pathways. Neuroscientists like to say that "cells that fire together wire together." Think of brain circuits like friendships: Those that are maintained and enriched will endure, while those that are neglected disappear.

Enriched environments are the key to optimal brain development. Laboratory animals provided with toys, companions, and more spacious living conditions grow additional brain cells. They also get smarter and perform better on behavioral tests such as wending their way through mazes. In humans, sensory and social deprivation early in life leads to decreases in intelligence, emotional health, and adaptation. But this dependence on the richness of environmental stimulation is not limited to early development. At every moment, your activities and your thoughts are modifying your brain. Intelligence is not something like eye color that you're born with and cannot change—it is a dynamic process that can be favorably influenced by choices you make.

Proper diet, exercise, and sleep are critical for optimal brain functioning. In general, what's good for the heart is good for the brain. By cutting down on empty calories in your diet, you can avoid obesity, which is now recognized as a risk factor for late-life dementia and other cognitive deficits. Research shows that regular exercise brings about positive changes in the brain function of children as well as adults. Simple, straightforward measures to improve sleep can also lead to big dividends at every age. More sleep, for instance, is characteristic of high-achieving students. Power naps can also help to enhance memory consolidation and cognitive performance.

Attention—also referred to as focus and concentration—must be rock solid in order to marshal the effort needed to improve your brain's performance. Attention in the mental sphere is the equivalent of endurance in the physical sphere. Just as an athlete cannot perform optimally without endurance, you cannot expect to achieve a superpower brain without being able to laser focus your mental energies. In order to do this, you must successfully manage 2 key factors in our current culture: distraction and multitasking. When you focus your attention on something, you have an easier time learning it and are more likely to remember it. The more you learn and the better you remember it, the greater your power to retrieve and use that information.

But if any piece of information can be instantly retrieved via a Google search, why bother to remember it? Because the act of remembering something facilitates the activation and retention of circuits within the brain that contribute to the brain's optimal functioning. Overreliance on electronic information aids can result in a disuse atrophy of your memory powers, but this atrophy can be overcome by deliberate efforts to improve memory. You'll learn how to enlist all of your senses in exercises and techniques that can enhance brain function in visual imagery, imagination, and long-term memory.

Working memory, also known as short-term memory, is the key to the most important mental operation carried out by the human brain: manipulating stored information. By improving your working memory, you can increase your intelligence as measured by standardized tests, along with such indirect measurements of intelligence as occupational achievement and creativity. Deliberate practice is the key to improving performance and creativity in all areas of human endeavor, including work and play.

Modern technology can be distracting, but it can be used to improve brain function. Think of technological aids as coextensions of your brain, capable of acting as brain boosters. A laptop computer, for instance, functions as a powerful and refined electronic extension of brain assistants dating back

2

to the earliest writing instruments. Video games, wisely used, can help you notice more, concentrate better, respond more quickly, and acquire specific real-world skills.

By challenging your brain to learn new information throughout your life, you build up cognitive reserve. This is analogous to monetary reserve: The more you have accumulated over your lifetime, the less susceptible you will be to deficits in your later years. In general, the more education and knowledge people acquire over their lifetime, the less likely they are in their later years to be diagnosed with dementia. In this practical course, you'll learn what steps you can take in your own life to enhance your brain function. ■

# How Your Brain Works
## Lecture 1

Listening to this lecture will change your brain. While you are hearing my words, your brain is shaping thoughts and images. You are remembering and associating what I'm saying with your experiences. You're forming new networks of ideas which are encoded in your brain's circuitry.

It was traditionally thought the brain was fully formed by adulthood, but in recent years neurobiologists have discovered that our brains continue to change throughout our lives, thanks to the phenomenon of plasticity. In this course we'll learn how you can take advantage of this exciting new research to optimize your brain fitness.

Let's look briefly at 3 of the important functions we'll explore in this course. The first is attention, which means focusing the mind on one thing at a time. Attention is the gateway to top-notch performance in math, reading, and auditory and visual memory. It is the coordinator of brain networks involving things like sensation, movement, emotions, and thinking. The second function is general memory. When we exercise our memory, we activate and maintain widely scattered circuits throughout the brain. In a future lecture we will discuss easy methods for developing a powerful memory. The third function is a special kind of memory: working memory. This is the most important mental operation carried out by the adult human brain. We use our working memory when we simultaneously keep multiple things "in mind" and mentally manipulate them.

As we'll see in later lectures, it's important to understand how to take advantage of the brain's various modes of processing and select the one that at any given moment is best. The more you learn about the brain, the greater your ability to apply meaningful exercises that will help you. Let's first cover a few basic principles of brain operation.

The frontal lobes are the CEO of the brain and the seat of controlled brain processing. They are linked with everything that distinguishes us from other animals, including foreseeing consequences of our actions, sequencing things, and executive control. But of course many of our actions aren't based on controlled processing: They occur on the basis of automatic processing. With automatic processing, choices are made with no sense of effort. Things just sort of happen, like walking across a room, eating a meal, or driving to the drugstore. When we encounter something unexpected and have to think about it or have to explain something to someone else, we shift to controlled processing.

Automatic processing is centered toward the back of the brain: the occipital, parietal, and temporal lobes. Controlled processing, however, mainly involves the anterior areas of the brain: the prefrontal and frontal areas. Cognition involves the whole brain and special senses—we have specific processes such as reading, writing, listening, or talking that we can't localize to one particular part of the brain. Emotions are a little bit more localizable: They involve deeper brain structures forming the limbic circuit and the right hemisphere. How does the brain manage to integrate our inner and outer experiences? As you may know, brain function is localized.

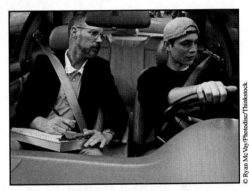

Driving can be done with automatic processing, but teaching someone else to drive demands controlled processing.

The right and left hemispheres each have different specializations, and each lobe in the hemispheres is concerned with specific processes. But despite the multiplicity of brain areas and functions, we experience the world as a unity.

Here's the key insight about how the brain works—information is the unit of exchange. It can range from the words you're reading now to the chemical exchanges occurring as each of your brain cells communicate with others. What about brain organization: Is the brain one vast interconnected fused

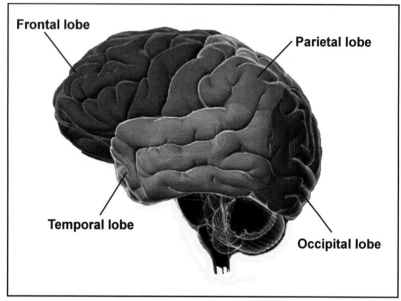

**The 4 lobes of the brain are associated with different functions.**

network of fibers, or are the nerve cells physically separated from each other? In fact, brain cells are connected similarly to how people on cell phones are connected. They're in touch with each other, but they're not physically connected. There can be strong or weak connections caused by distance, interference, and competing signals. In addition, there is entanglement: The neurons' branches are tightly entangled with each other. Think of the brain as a gigantic bowl of spaghetti, with each noodle highly branched and entangled but not quite physically connected with the others.

So far, we have learned that brain circuits and nerve cells can increase in number, and that each brain is the result of individual experiences and choices. The richer and more varied the experiences, the more enhanced the brain function. In other words, what you do shapes your brain's structure and function. We have also seen that the electrochemical activity in circuits determines their fate: "Cells that fire together, wire together." Information is widely disseminated among neurons, leading to higher-order processing such as memory, imagination, and creativity. The important thing is that the brain remains modifiable throughout our lives. In the next lecture, we'll learn more about our ability to change our brains through experience as we examine brain plasticity in more detail. ■

## Suggested Reading

Fields, *The Other Brain.*

LeDoux, *Synaptic Self.*

Purves, *Neuroscience.*

Purves et al., *Principles of Cognitive Neuroscience.*

## Questions to Consider

1. How might the brain processing involved in hitting a baseball differ from that of teaching someone to hit a baseball?

2. What are the capabilities and the limitations of brain imaging?

# How Your Brain Works
## Lecture 1—Transcript

Listening to this lecture will change your brain. While you are hearing my words your brain is shaping thoughts and images. You are remembering and associating what I'm saying with your experiences. You're forming new networks of ideas which are encoded in your brain's circuitry. Now this is very new because traditionally we thought the brain was fully-formed by adulthood, like all the other organs in our body. In fact, it is life experiences that shape and mold the brain throughout and influence neurotransmitters, which are the brain's messengers.

Hello, I'm Richard Restak, Clinical Professor of Neurology, George Washington University School of Medicine and Health Sciences. I've been studying and writing about the brain most of my adult life. My interest started in medical school and blossomed in recent years as neurobiologists discovered that our brains continue to change throughout our lives, thanks to what is called "plasticity." In this course we'll learn how you can take advantage of this exciting new research thought to optimize your brain fitness.

We'll explore how you can increase your brain's power by your own effort, apply what you learn about the brain to meet everyday challenges and enhance your quality of life, how to apply principles of brain operation to solve problems and learn new things. In addition to mental exercises, we'll examine the contribution of physical exercise to good brain health, we'll look at the importance of diet, the role of sleep and naps, we'll even have some fun with puzzles and games.

Here is a key point that we should set up from the very beginning: Physical and mental exercises differ. There is an important difference between strengthening the brain and improving general body conditioning. For instance if you practice any physical exercise it will lead to general health benefits such as decreased weight, blood pressure will lower, cholesterol will drop, increased stamina, and so forth.

Mental exercises, in contrast, tend to be more specific. For instance a memory exercise won't help you score higher on a test of logic, the bottom line is you will achieve the greatest benefit by working on separate functions such as visual observation, fine motor skills with your hands, tactile perception, logic, numbers, imagination, and visual-spatial thinking.

Let's look briefly at three of the important functions we'll explore in this course. The first is attention. By attention I mean focus keeping your mind on one thing at a time. The second is memory, general memory. And the third is a special kind of memory called, working memory. First: Attention. Attention is the gateway to topnotch performance in math, reading, and auditory and visual memory. It provides us with the basis for learning what to do and focus on and what to ignore. It is the coordinator of brain networks involving things like sensation, movement, emotions, and thinking.

The secondary is memory, which of course is an extension of attention. We can't use information we can't remember. When we exercise our memory we activate and maintain widely scattered circuits throughout the brain. In a future lecture we will discuss practical easy to learn methods for developing a super power memory. The third area is what's called working memory. This is the most important mental operation carried out by the adult human brain. Let me repeat that: This is the most important mental operation carried out by the adult human brain. We use our working memory when we simultaneously keep multiple things "in mind" and mentally manipulate them.

Let's cover a few basic principles of brain operation. Let's first start with the frontal lobes: the CEO of the brain and the seat of what's called controlled processing. The frontal lobes can be linked with everything that distinguishes us from other animals. Included here are: foreseeing consequences of our actions, sequencing things, executive control and drive. It's the frontal lobes that are involved whenever we consciously think something out, like preparing our income taxes getting all our expenses and income balanced out and thinking about what we're going to owe when we pay. This is what we mean by controlled processing. This usually means when we're talking about controlled processing, we are talking about thinking, we use words like "reasoning." Of course that this is much more "respectable" way of thinking because we've been led to believe that we are primarily "reasonable" creatures.

But of course many of our actions aren't based on controlled processing like reasoning, but occur on the basis of automatic processing: Things just "sort of happen" like my walking across a room, or eating a meal, or driving to the drugstore. With automatic processing choices are made with really no sense of effort. Typically they can't be easily explained to others. We're not even aware of how we decided. Now since consciousness isn't involved, our "reasoning" doesn't make it onto our mental radar screen. Let's talk a bit about the role of automatic processing in normal life: It's importance is that it frees up areas of the brain for other uses. Alfred North Whitehead, the philosopher, saw this and he stated that "Civilization advances by extending the number of operations that we can perform without thinking about them."

We shift to controlled processing when we encounter something unexpected and have to think about it or we have to explain something to someone else, teaching someone to drive is an example—it demands controlled processing. A balance, of course, is required: Too much automatic processing leads to impulsivity and simply act without reasoning or thinking. But too much controlled processing leads to a paralysis of indecision. We keep running over in our minds scenarios that we really can't make up our mind about what we're going to do.

Balance is also needed between cognitive and emotional brain processes. You'll hear a lot in these lectures about cognition, which is a fancy word, shorthand for all of our mental activities we use such as thinking, remembering, calculating, daydreaming, all of these responses that occur to our inner and outer worlds. As we will see in future lectures cognition and emotion often overlap. They're not so separate, many thoughts and experiences are accompanied by emotions. You pick up a telephone and it's the voice of an irritating sales call. Compare that to picking up the phone and it's the voice of a good friend. You're not just responding intellectually, you're responding emotionally to these two different experiences. The reasoning and emotional centers are linked in the brain.

Let's talk just a second about what brain areas are key for cognition and emotions and the distinction among them. Automatic processing is centered toward the back of the brain: occipital, parietal, and temporal lobes. Controlled processing however mainly involves the anterior areas of the brain: the prefrontal and frontal areas. Now cognition since it involves the whole brain and special senses, we have specific processes such as reading, writing, listening, talking, which we can't localize to one particular part of the brain. Emotions are a little bit more localizable, they involve deeper brain structures forming what's called the limbic circuit and the right hemisphere.

So how does the brain manage to integrate our inner and outer experiences? As you may already know, brain function is localized. We have the right and left hemispheres, and each of these have different specializations. Each lobe in the hemispheres is concerned with specific processes. But despite the multiplicity of brain areas and functions, we experience the world as a unity, as you are now as you're listening to this lecture it's all coming together as one unit. We experience what film-makers would refer to as scenarios: Sights and sounds and all other sensory inputs are synthesized into a unified experience, such as when you're driving to work—you're not hearing one thing or seeing one thing, it's all coming together into one total experience. Our understanding of how the brain binds our separate sensory inputs evolved actually from the early history of TV. Sound engineers worried that audio and video signals wouldn't synchronize. Then came the accidental discovery of a hundred millisecond window within the brain that automatically synchronizes the signals beyond that window—that narrow millisecond window—you have a badly dubbed movie. The brain automatically synthesizes sound and visual scenes into the unity of the movie that you are watching.

Here's a key insight about how the brain works—very insightful view that we're going to have about the information because information is the unit of exchange. Let me repeat that: Information is the unit of exchange. Messages are the token of informational exchange. Message transmission is the basic brain operation. Here's another key insight: "large brain reflects small brain." In other words, message transmission occurs at levels ranging from the easily observable (me talking to you) to the microscopic.

Now let's talk about brain organization, Is the brain one vast interconnected fused network of fibers? Or are the nerve cells physically separated from each other? The great deal of debate about this in the early 20th century, Ramon y Cajal, who was a neuroscience and also a great artist, felt that the brain cells were not in physical connection with each other, where as Camillo Golgidebate, who was an equally well-known neuroscientist, thought that it was like one essential net, one if you will spider web. Well no one was really sure who was correct. In fact the Nobel Prize committee of 1905 couldn't make up their mind who was correct and gave the Nobel prize to both of them.

In the interval special stains, special ways of staining neurons, revealed that neurons are separated from each other by a clasp or what's called a synapse, the axon of one cell is connected to another but it's not a physical connection. In fact brain cells are "connected" like people on cell phones are connected. They're in touch with each other but they're not physically connected. Also there can be strong or weak connections caused by distance, interference, competing signals, and so forth. In addition there is what's called entanglement: the neurons' branches are tightly entangled with each other. Think of the brain as a gigantic bowl of spaghetti with each noodle highly branched and entangled but not quite physically connected with others.

Message transmission between neurons takes place in 2 stages. The first is electrical: An electrical discharge is generated and travels along the length of an axon to the terminal at the synaptic space. The electrical signal then triggers the chemical stage, which is the release into the synapse of the neurotransmitter, which is the messenger molecule. The neurotransmitter enters the synapse and travels across like a ferryboat to receptors located on the membrane of the dendrite. Now what are receptors? Think of receptors are dynamic proteins within the cell membranes of the neuron we say "dynamic" because they can increase or decrease in number over very quick an short periods of time. For instance, an increase in number occurs in addiction, leading to a withdrawal reaction when the drug is unavailable: the receptors "cry out for the chemical" the withdrawal reaction ends when the receptors decrease in number.

Well let's get back to the ferryboat trip. The ferryboat trip from pre to postsynaptic neuron takes one thousandth of a second. Each neurotransmitter attaches to a special receptor just like a lock would attach to a key, highly specific. One dendritic cell then another is activated or inhibited from firing. At this point communication reverts again to an electric signal which travels along that axon until reaching the next terminal where communication becomes chemical once again. It's a life cycle for neurotransmitters of after attaching to the dendritic membrane the neurotransmitters are either reabsorbed by the presynaptic neuron and prepared for re-release or they're broken down into smaller chemicals. Think of the brain as the summation of billions of interacting neurons influencing each other via the interplay of hundreds of neurotransmitters and their receptors.

Now let's shift our focus from the molecular world of neurotransmitters and receptors to the scale of the whole brain. The brain is the organ that during my neurology training I've even held in my hands. It's possible to discern a history of our understanding of the brain and physicians learned about the abnormal brain. That's because early research tools were dangerous to use in normal people, so neuroscientists learned about the brain from people with brain damage. Of course, learning about deficits does help to understand normal function but only up to a point. Now, thanks to newer safer imaging methods, neuroscientists can carry out wide ranging studies of the brain's processing in everyday life.

We have to think about it in 2 ways called structural imaging and process imaging. When we talk about structural imaging think carpenter; it shows the location where things are happening. A CAT scan or MRI or magnetic resonance imaging as it's called, is an example of structural imaging. For process imaging think electrician, activities. Process imaging shows electrochemical activity, that's things like fMRI and PET. We have methods that illustrate shifts in neurotransmitters, ions, and magnetic fields.

Now imaging is good, it can do a lot but it can't do everything. Let's talk about what it can do: It can measure blood flow which increases as neurons become active and we get what we call activation maps. If you did one right now it would show parts of my brain that have the activation of thinking, my lips, my tongue, my hands, all that's activated. You'd see an activation pattern of someone speaking. If we did an activation pattern of your brain it'd be someone listening to something and thinking about what they're hearing. Activation maps can do other things such as serve as a marker for diseased states, we mentioned addiction a few moments ago. It can also provide developmental profiles such as adolescence, you can tell probably how old someone is within certain ranges by looking at the imaging.

Now imaging can't do certain things. It can't predict individual behavior or proclivities, it can't say someone is going to turn out this way or that way on the basis of a brain image. And it can't always optimize current treatments for brain disorders. Remember the individual regions work independently and come together.

In addition, the more abstract the concept the harder it is to localize it on a brain image. Take courage for instance. There's no area of the brain that's going to light up for courage or consciousness. This was what we think of as "neuromythology." It's a little bit like in the 19th and early 20th centuries they talked about phrenology that one could tell what someone was thinking by looking at a part of the brain and how big it was, or how big that part of the skull was. We know now that something like that just doesn't hold up.

Here's some basic brain facts, some numbers to take in that are just truly extraordinary. The brain encompasses 100 billion neurons with each neuron connected to perhaps 10,000 others for a total of 1 million billion connections. Wow, it's hard to get a mental picture of a number like 1 million billion so let's sneak up on it in stages. A million is easy: $1000 \times 1000$ about the size of a small city. A billion is $1000 \times 1$ million, which is the size of 1000 small cities or 100 very large cities. Now to put 1 million billion in perspective, there are about 6 billion people currently living on our planet, which is a small number compared to those 100 billion nerve cells and a truly paltry number compared to those 1 million billion connections. Also consider the difficulty in tracing the nerve cell connections. The lowly worm C. elegans has a brain contains 300 neurons, so we're really way down there compared to what we talked about a second ago, and this has 7000 synapses. So 300 neurons and 7000 synapses, sounds like the easiest thing. Actually manually tracing the connections without the help of a computer took 10 years to complete.

In comparison let's look at another simulation of nerve cell birth and growth, and this time we're going to talk about the human brain. Now this video that you're looking at focuses on the dynamism of what's happening in a small section of the brain. It shows an interlacing of the neuronal fibers. It shows a vast interconnectivity at all levels. And the bottom line here is what you do affects dynamic processes like this in your own brain, this is also the underlying theme of this course. This video gives you an example of why even computers will have difficulty tracing the neuron connections in the human brain. Sorry to say there isn't a quick solution to the numbers problem. Sebastian Seung, who had something to do with the film we're watching now, is professor of Computational Neuroscience at MIT and he has this to say about human brain tracing: "You would need 100 million terabytes to store the images from the human brain. Even with 10,000 microscopes working in parallel, it might take 30 years to collect all the images. Analyzing the images could require a parallel supercomputer with millions of processors." Here is the dilemma: Computer counting results in many mistakes and computers they're not always reliable and can't accurately "see" the shape of the neurons because the neurons do vary considerably in shape. Manual tracing is incredibly time consuming, even for a cubic millimeter of brain tissue, as we saw in this video. Here's the take-home message: Don't expect to see a wiring diagram of the human brain in your lifetime.

Let's turn to brain development. The neurons are produced first followed by synapse, which makes sense since you can't have a synapse connecting one neuron to another until you have some neurons. Synaptic connections form rapidly. In fact in the womb, they're coming in at a million per second. In the first month of life synapses increase from 50 trillion to 1 quadrillion, back again to these incredible numbers. Unused synapses are eliminated by pruning which results in more efficient circuits—and pruning is just like you would think about in a garden you go out there and get rid of things that aren't working, nothing's happening, they're gone. Now there are patterns of brain growth: There's a linear and progressive increase in brain weight, volume, and head size. Increasing numbers of synapses also come until a plateau is reached followed by a decrease in nerve cells determined by usage and circuitry formation.

The total brain volume peaks at age 11 in girls and 15 in boys. Male brain on average, now we're talking on the average, is 10% larger. Brain reaches maximum weight by early adulthood and decreases 10% over the lifespan. Think of a 3 pound organ with 100 million nerve cells and a million billion synapses; it undergoes functional changes over the lifetime. Between 3 to 6 months the brain achieves its maximum brain cell number. From 7 months to 2 years nerve cell numbers decrease while connections, or synapses, increase.

Forty percent of synapses generated in infancy are lost by adulthood: This is the "use it or lose it" theme which goes throughout the whole study of the brain, those parts of the brain that are not used are endanger of being eliminated. The brains of animals with enriched environments contain 25% more synapses, and we're going to go into that in the next lecture with more about this in lecture two on plasticity.

There's also patterns of brain growth with distinct peaks occurring at certain times such as age 3, when you have individuation; age 7 the beginning of concrete reasoning starts; ages 11 and 12 when you have the influence of hormones and the onset of puberty; At age of 15 when abstract reasoning and judgment starts when a person is thought to have legal responsibility for their actions. Beyond 15, brain development depends very much on experience.

With maturation grey matter, or brain cells, decreases, white matter, or the connections, increases. Myelination, which is a term for insulation, of white matter progresses from inferior to superior and from posterior to anterior. The white matter increase is associated with greater efficiency and speed of conduction. Particularly important with the frontal cortex and cerebellum which mature late-there are intimate connections between these two. Let's talk now about the cerebral cortex, which is the outer of the brain. If you take a deck of cards and take out 6 cards, there are essentially 2mm in thickness and they have 6 layers. Each one is different, each one is interconnected. That's what we're seeing with the brain; it has the same arrangement. To appreciate this, just think about that. You can use business cards as well, or as I did a deck of cards. Now stretched out the human cortical sheet, which is what we're talking about, is about the size of a large dinner napkin. The monkey neocortical sheet is the size of a business envelope. Beneath the cerebral cortex is the white matter, which is tightly bundled communication lines linking points in the brain. Think of the tightly wound fibers of a baseball that are hidden beneath the leather covering, in this case the leather covering is the cortical mantle.

Within this bundle of white fibers are the glial cells. The classical view was that the glial cells constituted a "scaffolding" for neurons, glia means "glue" in Greek. Glia cells outnumber neurons by as much as 6 to 1 in parts of the brain. So obviously the brain is more complicated than we imagined even a few years ago. Neurons at 100 billion are outnumbered by glial cells, and we're not certain at this point of all the functions of the glial cells is. They process information we know that, but they do it differently than neurons. They're slower and they communicate it broadly rather than linearly. We have a new concept of glial cells which are now known to be involved in message transmission and reception. They don't generate electrical impulses but they do respond to them. They use calcium ions instead of electrical signals. And they possess sensors that detect signaling by neurons and they can alter it.

Next let's say a few words about the basal ganglia, which are islands of grey matter suspended in the white matter, so they're down underneath these islands that are connected to each other and they're connected to the cerebral cortex. The frontal cortex particularly is especially interconnected with the basal ganglia. They're concerned with organizing automatic rather than intentionally directed behavior, as I walk across the room for instance I have something in mind, to pick up something, that's the frontal cortex. When I went to get those cards for instance, the frontal cortex set that up. But each move that I made was not being controlled or thought out. So these circuits are extremely complex and convoluted with both positive and negative effects.

The brain is a work in progress, which is a new insight. New neurons are created over the lifespan. We have granule cells in hippocampus and the dentate gyrus continue to be produced. That's called neurogenesis which can be increased by enriched environments or inhibited by stress, depression, sleep deprivation, anxiety, things like this.

We also have an experience-dependent brain. Infants are born with the capacity to perceive and react to the phonemes of all the languages in the world, whatever language they here they can react to it. By 6 months this capacity is lost. For instance if Japanese children if they don't hear English they lose the ability to make the distinction between "r" and "l" sounds. Exposure to language increases proficiency: 20 month olds with a talkative mom know 130 more words than a child with a laconic mom. At age 2 the number has risen to 300 words. Only live interaction with a person works, not live TV. The child's 3rd grade achievement is related to the amount of early language exposure, so you can see the importance of this.

We have critical and sensitive periods. Kittens deprived of vision in first 3 months of life for instance, grow up with permanent visual impairments. Songbirds that do not hear their native sounds cannot produce those sounds. Monkeys raised in isolation grow up with emotional problems. Among people with "perfect pitch" this occurs only in musicians who started training before age 7. In order to speak a foreign language without an accent a child must speak the language's phonemes by puberty. But despite these sensitive periods or critical windows, the brain is still able to form some new connections and new associations not only in adulthood but far into old age.

So, what have we learned so far? Brain circuits and nerve cells can increase in number. Each brain is the result of individual experiences and choices. The richer, the more varied the experiences the more enhanced the brain function. In other words, what you do shapes your brain's structure and function. The electrochemical activity in circuits determines their fate. We say "cells that fire together wire together." Information is widely disseminated among neurons leading to higher order processing such as memory, imagination, and creativity. The important thing is that the brain remains modifiable throughout our lives.

In the next lecture we'll learn more about our ability change our brains through experience as we examine brain plasticity in more detail. Thank you.

# How Your Brain Changes
## Lecture 2

Technology can also bring about changes in the brain thanks to plasticity. Our widespread use of Internet-based technologies leads to changes in our thinking patterns involving superficial approaches to knowledge: scanning, skimming, "idea shopping," browsing, and multitasking.

Now that we've learned something about how your brain is organized, let's talk about how changes in your brain can improve the way you function in day-to-day life. Intelligence was traditionally considered to be fixed—something we're born with, like eye color. But there has been a revolutionary transformation in our thinking: Intelligence is not a fixed trait but can be modified over a lifespan. James Flynn, an intelligence researcher at the University of Otago in Dunedin, New Zealand, demonstrated that from 1947 to 2002, Americans gained 24 points on testing for similarities but only 4 points on vocabulary and 2 points on math. Why was there such a gain only in similarities? It is because we're using our intelligence in different ways. We have more education and more leisure activities, and in the process we have altered the balance between the abstract and the concrete.

Brain research was revolutionized by the discovery of plasticity, the science of which is simple: (1) When you exercise your brain, you release natural growth factors and influence neurotransmitters, which enhance your brain's level of performance. (2) The efficiency of cell-to-cell communication via chemical messengers increases. (3) There is a remapping of the functional connections among neurons, as new things are learned new maps are created, or old maps altered. (4) Alternative circuits can be established to compensate for lost or injured areas.

Circuits and networks—not the number of nerve cells—are the key to improved function. Learning is the means of establishing and maintaining these circuits. Think of brain circuits like friendships: Those that are maintained and enriched will endure; those that are neglected will disappear.

Maintenance, novelty, and enriched experiences are like fertilizer on the brain and bring about growth and development

How do we know this? Here is a human example of enriched experience. If you have been to London and taken cabs, you have seen that London cab drivers really know the city. You tell them where you want to go, and they don't have to consult anything—they take you right there. That's not by accident: They study the streets of London for 2 years and take a competitive test for their job. Not surprisingly, a study of London cab drivers shows that they have a larger than average hippocampus, with size related to years of driving experience.

In this lecture we have talked about 2 main points: Your brain and your intelligence can change throughout your lifespan. And most important, you are able to shape those changes in your own brain. In the next lecture, we'll move from plasticity to the importance for brain health of what you eat, how you exercise, and how well you sleep. ∎

## Plasticity-Enhancing Exercises

We often pay insufficient attention to what our senses are telling us, so it is helpful to exercise our elementary physical sensations. There are 3 types of exercises I'd like you to practice: visual and auditory exercises, sensory and motor exercises involving hand dexterity, and peripersonal space exercises. Here are a few examples for you to try.

**Visual exercises.** Actors have always used sense memory, which they have traditionally practiced with a coffee cup. Give it a try: Hold the cup; recognize and memorize its height, its color, its composition; any ridges or design it has; and light reflections. Now involve your other senses: How does it feel? How heavy is it? You are trying to re-create the cup in your brain. The same brain circuits are involved as when dealing with exploring the real cup. An actor can make the audience "see" a cup that he's not actually holding because of this ability. Pick any other object that interests you, and re-create it via a similar exercise.

**Auditory exercises.** In the 1950s, Jack Foley at Universal Pictures came up with the idea of assembling a studio where he could create live sound effects for movies by using simple and readily available sources. This required a sharp ear for sounds—for instance, crumpling a newspaper sounds like fire. Try it for yourself. Close your eyes, roll a newspaper up, put it to your ear, and crumple it. It sounds just like a fire. Foley artists need a sharp ear for the sounds of everyday objects to create their special effects. For instance, the laser blasts in *Star Wars* were made by taking a hammer and hitting a high-tension wire that supports an antenna. As a sound exercise, listen to the things around you in order to sharpen your sensitivity. Try to figure out what sounds might be substituted for others.

**Motor exercises.** Exercises involving the hand are functionally related to the brain. Developing nimble fingers is a surefire way of improving brain function: Take up juggling or a hobby that requires fine detail work like knitting, painting, or drawing.

**Peripersonal space exercises.** These exercises have to do with a virtual envelope around the skin's surface that extends our body boundaries. Try this exercise: Move your hands toward each other so that your fingers touch. It's not very hard to do. But try it with your eyes closed, and you'll find that it's difficult because you don't have much experience doing it. You're not initially able to do well because of your brain's overreliance on vision. Take up a sport that demands an awareness of your body boundary and its extensions. Tennis is a good example: You have to know where your arm is, where you're standing, and how to correlate exactly where to place the ball so it's just within the court. This type of exercise will help you achieve an enhanced kinesthetic sense.

## Suggested Reading

Fields, *The Other Brain.*

LeDoux, *Synaptic Self.*

Nisbett, *Intelligence and How to Get It.*

Purves, *Neuroscience.*

Purves et al., *Principles of Cognitive Neuroscience.*

Restak, *Mozart's Brain and the Fighter Pilot.*

Schwartz and Begley, *The Mind and the Brain.*

# How Your Brain Changes
## Lecture 2—Transcript

Welcome to Lecture 2 on how your brain changes. Now that we've learned something about how your brain is organized, let's talk about how changes in your brain can improve the way you function in day to day life. For instance intelligence: Traditionally we considered intelligence to be fixed and unmodifiable, something we're born with, like eye color. Now comes a revolutionary transformation in our thinking: intelligence is not a fixed trait but can be modified over a lifetime. It changes as our brains change. I'm referring here to the findings of James Flynn, an intelligence researcher at the University of Otago in Dunedin, New Zealand. Flynn demonstrated that from 1947 to 2002, Americans gained 24 points on IQ tests for similarities but only 4 points on vocabulary and 2 points on math. Why such a gain only in similarities? That's because we're using our intelligence differently ways. Now we have more education and more leisure activities, and in the process we have altered the balance between the abstract and the concrete. In agrarian and hunter societies intelligence over hundreds of years, intelligence was practical and literal talking about growth and talking about animals, and trails and things like that. But thanks to urbanization, education and the permeation of scientific thinking into our everyday lives, we now can move beyond thinking only about the "here and now." We can actually work with concepts that involve abstraction.

Intelligence today involves the ability to think outside the bounds of personal observation and experience. Proverbs are good examples of this "A rolling stone gathers no moss," it's really not about stones or about moss, it's about that one has to keep moving along in order to prosper and do well. "A stitch in time save nine" is not about stitches or time or nine, it's about taking precautions to make sure bad things don't happen. "People in glass houses shouldn't throw stones" means that you shouldn't criticize people for things that actually refer to yourself as well. Now here's a hard one you can think about yourself in your own time: "The tongue is the enemy of the neck."

How did this change come about from literal experienced based thinking to abstract thinking? Let's discover and discuss whether it can be entirely explained by genetics? Flynn thought genetic changes could not account for the increase; there simply isn't enough time. Instead, intelligence is related to cultural forces and it can change in tandem with these changes. Now this deals a death blow to the theory that our cognitive powers are dependent on genetic factors alone. For one thing, twin studies favoring genetics are flawed. Flynn uses an interesting analogy taken from basketball. Imagine 2 twins separated at birth, tall both of them are very tall, and both of them have no initial interest in basketball but because they're tall basketball players would approach them and ask "Have you ever thought about playing basketball?" That got them into the basketball circuit, and soon they'll be in the NBA. As Flynn says "there is a strong tendency for a genetic advantage (such as tallness) to get more and more matched to a corresponding environment." Flynn concluded that the environment plays a great role in enhancing our cognitive powers. We can further this goal through our efforts such as what we learn and what we do. For instance, we can increase our intelligence by solving math problems, interpreting literature, finding on-the-spot solutions to problems, assimilating the scientific worldview, and trying to practice some wisdom. Most important is to seek challenging cognitive environments.

As an example, let me tell you about Rachel. When Rachel was born and tested later, about age 7 or 8, she was found to have an average I.Q. But she was born into a home where parents provided intellectually stimulating experiences such as books, and when she fell behind she had tutors who helped her with those subjects. The parents remained involved but not over-involved with school and teachers, in other words, they weren't what we call "helicopter parents." Now thanks to these efforts Rachel was accepted into a superior high school. Once there she had to work harder but she did well. She graduated in the top 20% of her class. As a result of that she was accepted into small well-regarded university. While there she met a teacher who inspired her to be a lawyer and to work hard and try to get into a law school, which she did. And after law school she joined a firm specializing in intellectual property. While there she met and married a colleague who combines his legal career with music and plays in a jazz group. Now Rachel and her husband are involved in all sorts of cultural activities where they're living. The bottom line is that Rachel's experiences have taken her further than her modest I.Q. would have predicted. Her environment outpaced her genetic inheritance as a determinant of her achievement.

Now what's going on in the brain that could account for these changes? As I mentioned in the last lecture, brain research was revolutionized by the discovery of what we call "plasticity." Incidentally when I say plasticity and talk about plasticity I don't mean plastic bottles and things like that, there's a big difference between plastic and plasticity. By plasticity I mean something that is malleable. The science of plasticity and potential for growth is simply explained: When you exercise your brain, you release natural growth factors like brain-derived neurotropic factor BDNF (BDNF) and you also influence neurotransmitters, which enhance your brain's level of performance. Plasticity refers to all of the changes and things that can change in the structure and/or function of the brain such as neurogenesis, which is the brain's ability to add new nerve cells. That's a new concept by the way, use to be thought that there were never new brain cells, now we know that there are, at least in parts of the hippocampus. Secondly there's increases in the efficiency of cell to cell communication via chemical messengers. Third we have a remapping of the functional connections among neurons, as new things are learned new maps are created, or old maps altered. Fourth we have the establishment of alternative circuits to compensate for lost or injured areas, for instance after a stroke a person may not be able to more their right arm. If you constrain that arm in a sling and force them to use their left hand and arm you'll begin to get improvement. Much of what we've learned about plasticity comes from animal research in enriched environments. William Greenough of the University of Illinois at Champaign-Urbana worked in 1970s with two groups of rats. One group of rats was in what we would call "lockdown," they're isolated, they didn't have any contact with other rats, they didn't have anything stimulating, nothing happening all day long. The second group was in what Greenough called the rat equivalent of Disneyland, they had toys, and wheels, and other rats, and interactions and things like that. They were more socially and physically active. The toys, brighter cages, network and coexisting with other rats.

Under the microscope 25% more synapses per neuron were found in second group of the enriched rats. They had a greater brain volume; they had improved learning, and best of all, this correlation continued across their lifespan. Take home message: If you want to make a rat grow up smarter, make its life more challenging, increase its opportunities for sensory stimulation, physical exercise, and socialization. Each of these enhances the brain's development and leads to smarter rats. My thoughts on Greenough studies as a matter of fact, think about it for a moment—even "enriched" rats in a lab are deprived compared to rats in natural environment, which have to deal with predators and wander their way through very complicated mazes for food. So the enriched "laboratory environment" doesn't really nearly correspond to what the rat would find in the natural environment. So the enriched laboratory environment was what the study was about. The tantalizing question is: Would an enriched environment in the real world lead to enhancement in the human brain?

Let me tell you about the Bucharest early intervention project. It compared abandoned children reared in institutions to abandoned children moved from the institutions to be raised in foster care. Their cognitive development was tracked through 54 months. The children who remained in institutions remained far below the children removed to foster care. The younger the child when placed in foster care, the better the result. Now this suggests a sensitive period during the first 2 years of life when the brain is especially vulnerable, recall that as we mentioned the brain is plastic and will be shaped according to experience. If you enrich that experience and the brain thrives.

Environmental enrichment not limited to infancy. Let me tell you about a recent study on dyslexia. As you know dyslexia has to do with difficulty in reading. It's a lifelong problem but it's not necessarily associated with I.Q. or achievement. My medical school roommate was dyslexic but still graduated near the top of the class. Years later on a book tour I gave him a copy of one of my book. He looked at it and smiled and said "Thank a lot but you know I'll never read it." He was making a point that dyslexics do not read for pleasure, they just read for practical reasons. Marcel Just and Tim Keller of Carnegie Mellon carried out a research project involving dyslexic children between age 8 and 10. They introduced a reading remediation program lasting only 6 months but it led to an increase in white matter in the areas of the brain responsible for language. Thirty seven poor readers received remedial instruction, while 12 did not. The white matter changes occurred only in the remedial group. Anatomical changes, incidentally, coincided with the improvements in reading. This is what's called a brain-behavior correlation, a change in brain structure or function corresponding to a behavioral change.

The explanation of the dyslexia results are repeated use of circuits stimulated oligodendrocytes to produce more myelin along the axons being fired, this increases speed of conduction. Even modest modifications in white matter may enable major changes in cognitive ability, as Just and Keller claim and wrote in their Neuron paper. According to Dr. Just this study provided evidence that repeated cognitive exercises can alter the connectivity of the human brain. This course is based on that insight. In a later lecture we will be talking about a form of repeated cognitive exercise called intensive deliberate practice. The main theme is repeated cognitive exercises lead to mastery and to changes in the brain. For instance intense piano practice increases white matter but according to the intensity of practice. A little bit of practice, little bit of change; a lot of practice a lot of change in the white matter.

We are dealing here with a fundamental principle. We sculpt our brains according to our life experiences. No two brains are alike not even the brains of identical twins. Using imaging you can even make inferences about a person based on his or her brain organization. A skilled pianist shows activation in the brain's finger areas while listening to music or watching someone else perform music, but he shows no response when watching random finger movements over a keyboard. A similar activation occurs in the relevant brain areas in ballet dancers and surgeons. We speak here of "brain memory" you've often heard the word "muscle memory" but it's not the "muscle memory" it's "brain memory."

Think of human brain development as existing on a continuum across the lifespan. Brains at all ages share the same challenges: need for stimulation, the need to maintain nerve cell circuits despite a steady loss of neurons. There is also a striking paradox here that's worth mentioning, mainly that improved function comes about with fewer components. The brain is unlike any other biological or mechanical structure. Imagine buying a car that after 6 months you pull the hood up and take a part out and it would run better, better mileage, better gas use and so forth. Well that would be a very strange car, but yet the brain works that way. The maximum brain cell number between 3 and 6 months of age before we are born. During the next 3 months before birth, and continuing during first 2 years of life, the number of neurons decreases even more while functional connections, or synapses, increase. This corresponds to change in grey/white matter ratio, think of the brain as being sculpted by experience. Now keep in mind an infant at birth has fewer neurons than during later part of gestation, but a far greater number than it will have as an adult. We refer to this as pruning. Those of you who do gardening know what I mean by this, you go out and you cut off branches that aren't healthy and you just keep those that are viable.

Circuits and networks not nerve cell numbers are the key to improved function. Learning is the means of establishing and maintaining these circuits. For instance reading remediation is an example as with the Just and Keller research I mentioned a moment ago. Think of brain circuits like friendships: Those that are maintained and enriched will endure; those that are neglected will disappear. Maintenance, novelty, enriched experiences are like fertilizer on the brain and they bring about growth and development.

How do we know this? Here are some human examples of enriched experience. Those of you that have been to London and taken cabs have seen that the London cab drivers really know the city. You tell them where you want to go, and they don't have to consult anything they take you right there. That's not just by accident they studied for 2 years all the streets of London and they've taken a competitive test for it. Well a study of the London cab drivers shows that they have a larger hippocampus with size related to years of driving experience. So that's all encoded in this hippocampus. One wonders what the effect will be of GPS, which at some point will be introduced? I speculate a decrease in hippocampus size.

The second example is a study of older adults learning to juggle 3 balls over 3 months. It showed an increase volume visual cortex, the hippocampus, and the nucleus accumbens. These changes disappeared 3 months after juggling stopped. A third example is a sighted person can be taught by wearing a blindfold after 10 minutes of practice that he can acquire the skill of a person that is blind in the use of a cane. That's what's called an enlargement of peripersonal space. Now that awareness disappears after only a few minutes when the blindfold is removed. Notice the short time span involved: only 10 minutes.

We create new patterns of brain organization based on what we see, what we do, what we imagine, and what we learn. Learning something new establishes pathways consisting of millions of brain cells. Now doing and not just observing is what is important. We have to activate what is called the action-observation network. Remember the experience of ballet dancers I mentioned earlier, the development of "muscle memory" which is really brain memory? This is based on what's called the simulation hypothesis, the use of motor memory to interpret what other people are doing. Skilled athletes can watch and predict another athlete's performance, boxers are particularly good at this. A professional boxer once told me he can see the punch coming before the person throwing it even knows what they're going to do.

All of these examples are based on mirror neurons in the prefrontal cortex. These are a cluster of cells originally observed in the macaque monkey. The cells respond when one monkey watches another one grasp a peanut. These are the same cells that respond when the monkey grasps the peanut itself. Mirror neurons are task specific; they work according to what's called a perception-action matching system. If you watch me reach for a cup of tea, your brain becomes active in the same areas that are used when I'm reaching for that cup of tea. But if I reach for the tea cup for another reason or in another situation, such as cleaning up after a tea party, nothing happens. The mirror neuron's are not activated.

Now let's talk about the body image and its alterations. What is body image? Well look at pictures or videos of yourself taken at different ages, when you're 8 or 10 years of age. Your image of yourself and what your body was like is certainly different than it is now. It can be altered subtly; a new hairstyle or clothing outfit can also change your body image. The body image can also expand to include things that are external to ourselves. Parking space lines, for instance, look smaller to Hummer drivers compared to Prius drivers. The extension of body boundaries include attachment to electronic gadgets. You'll often notice that when you buy something electronic you have to have it repaired or replaced at the manufacturers discretion. That's because we can become very attached, it can become part of our body image. We're also aware of things like "you're in my space" feeling that our body boundary is being violate. One driver is cut off for instance on the road and sets of an episode of road rage because they're body image and body space has been invaded. Great cultural differences exist concerning how close other people should be lest they become offensive .

Let's talk about Learning: think of the branching of a tree. In full bloom, the tree gives off branches, twigs, leaves, and blossoms. Similarly, learning leads to fuller and richer circuits; if learning stops the brain reverts to a state similar to the tree in winter: bare branches, no leaves, stark, and skeletal. Remember: Learning is specific. A ballet dancers' brain responds when watching other ballet dancers, but does not respond to ballroom dancers. We sculpt our brain and our learning by our specific experiences. Surgeons have greater activation in the hand areas of the brain compared to non-surgeons. Perhaps that why many retired surgeons take up hobbies related to finger agility such as cut glass and ceramics. All of these professions have shaped their brains by virtue of their experience.

Technology can also bring about changes in the brain thanks to plasticity. Our widespread use of Internet-based technologies leads to changes in our thinking patterns, like scanning, skimming, "idea shopping," browsing, and multitasking. In the lecture on technology we will examine in more detail the effect of technology on our cognition including why technology rather than biology will determine future brain development. In fact it already has: the thinking patterns of the "web generation" differ from the traditional ways of obtaining information.

In the last part of this lecture I want to suggest some plasticity enhancing exercises. We will start with elementary physical sensations because we often pay insufficient attention to what our senses are telling us. This leads to failures of memory: we can't remember what we never registered. We're going to talk about 3 exercises: visual and auditory exercises, sensory and motor exercises involving hand dexterity, and peripersonal space exercises.

First visual exercises. Actors have always used sense-memory. A traditional one is the use of a coffee cup—an empty coffee cup. You hold one; you recognize its height, its color, its composition, the ridges on lips, artwork, design—and you're memorizing this—light reflections. When finished looking at it, involve your other senses. How does it feel? How sound does it make when flick it on the edge? How heavy is it? The goal is to recreate the cup in your brain. The same brain circuits are involved incidentally as when dealing with exploring the real cup. An actor can make audience "see" a cup that he's not actually holding because of this ability to actually make everything look just right like he's holding a cup. Now you can take any object that interests you, doesn't have to be a coffee cup, and recreate it via a similar exercise.

Sound exercises involve paying attention to the sounds around you. Here's an example: In the 1950s Jack Foley a film editor at Universal Pictures came up with the idea of assembling a studio where he could create live sound effects for movies by using simple and readily available sources. This required a sharp ear for sounds, for instance crumpling a newspaper sounds like fire. Try it for yourself. Close your eyes, get a newspaper, roll it up and put it to your ear and crumple it. It sounds just like a fire. Foley artists need a sharp ear for the sounds of everyday objects to create their special effects. For instance, the laser blasts in *Star Wars* were made by taking a hammer and hitting a high tension wire that supports an antenna. Stabbing a body is essentially like the sound of a knife stabbing a watermelon. The sound of bone crushing can be made by crunching celery. As a sound exercise: Listen to the things around you in order to sharpen your sensitivity. Try to figure out what sounds might be substituted for others.

You can use classical music: compare composers, performers. and performances. Or take your own special interests; some people are interested in the sounds of certain birds and correlating them to pictures or seeing the birds. In one personal example, at my home in Prince Edward Island in the summer there are a lot of frogs and I've sort of come to recognize the call of different frogs from listening to them and listening to different recordings. There's another area of listening that's important and that's for emotions in human voices. The human voice has a lot of leakage of emotions because of changes in tone, cadence, loudness, and pacing.

Exercises involving the hand are functionally related to the brain, it's very important. A large area of the brains is showing the hand, correlated to the hand. Developing "nimble fingers" is a surefire way of improving brain function. Take up juggling or a hobby that requires fine detail work like knitting, painting, drawing, manipulating or penmanship. I have a great interest in pens because I try to improve my cursive writing.

Exercises of peripersonal space have to do with a virtual envelope around the skin's surface that extends our body boundaries. For instance try this exercise, just take your fingers and move them forward so they touch. It's not very hard to do, but try it with your eyes closed and you'll find that it's actually difficult to do because we don't really have much experience doing it. Another thing to do is to pretend that you've got a gun and pointing it at your toe. No problem as long as your eyes are open but when you do it with your eyes closed you're not able to do it as well. You're not initially able to do well because of your brain's over-reliance on vision. Take up a sport that demands an awareness of your body boundary and its extensions. Tennis is a good example, you have to know where your arm is, where you're standing, you have to know about the ball, you have to be able to just correlate exactly where you're going to have to place it so it's just within the court and not outside and an illegal shot. If you do this you will achieve an enhanced kinesthetic sense. Kinesthetic sense exercises are performed all the time by musicians and athletes as they work toward is making up what we call embodied knowledge. To be able to take what they've learned and be able to make it almost automatic; it becomes part of the body image that we've been talking about.

I think the very best is tai chi. I've done this for years and tai chi you learn this complicated form, it takes a while to learn it but it's worth doing, and after that you're able to realize where parts of your body are when you're making a certain movement. A good teacher will ask you to close your eyes and image where your arm is, and then you imagine it, and then you look and it takes a while to develop the ability to know exactly where your hand and arm is.

In the lecture on sensory memory, I will describe additional exercises involving touch and the special senses of taste and smell. So in this lecture we have talked about 2 main points. Your brain and your intelligence can change throughout your lifespan. And most importantly, you are able to shape those changes in your own brain. In the next lecture, we'll move from plasticity to the importance for brain health of what you eat, how you exercise, and how well you sleep. We'll talk about that next time.

# Care and Feeding of the Brain
## Lecture 3

**Older adults with a history of exercise have better-preserved brains than those who have not exercised.**

There are 3 prongs to the care and feeding of the brain: diet, sleep, and exercise. First we examine diet. Obesity is cognitively harmful, and controlling your weight is a way of improving your brain. But how much caloric restriction is necessary? The class of foods chosen is less important than the number of calories eaten. Sixty-five years of animal research shows that the rate of degenerative disease is slowed by caloric restriction, which means a balanced reduction of protein, fat, and carbs without reduction of nutrient content. It's been shown that animals that eat 35% fewer calories live 35% longer. They are also healthier and have enhanced cognitive performance.

Would a severely decreased caloric diet work in humans as well? A National Institute of Aging study showed that a 25% caloric restriction resulted in a lowering of body temperature and insulin levels, which suggests that such a diet might work. But a key issue here is that few people would be willing to conform to such a diet. Fortunately, keeping calories low enough to prevent obesity may be sufficient.

Let's explore the harmful cognitive effects of obesity. Animal research shows that diets high in saturated fats lead to animals' underperformance on tests of memory and tests of reinforcing rewards (e.g., pressing a button to get food). Similar effects are likely in humans—reduction in fats and "empty calories" will improve memory and brain function. A new insight is that addiction and obesity are linked together. High-fat, high-calorie diets decrease the responsiveness of the brain's pleasure centers. Changes in brain chemistry involving dopamine and opioids lead to compulsive eating patterns. Obesity and addiction may result from similar maladaptations in the brain's reward systems.

The bottom line is that eliminating obesity isn't always easy, but it is worth the effort because of the effects on the brain. Start by eliminating from your diet those foods that can be proven to cause harm. First eliminate trans fats—fats that are formed when liquid oils are transformed into solid fats by adding hydrogen to vegetable oil. Avoid hydrogenated and partially hydrogenated foods. Fast foods are the worst: fried chicken, fried fish, biscuits, French fries, potato chips, doughnuts, and muffins. Substitute them in your diet with fruits, vegetables, chicken, whole-grain breads, and green leafy vegetables.

Another important food source is omega-3 unsaturated fatty acids. They're found in oily fish like mackerel, salmon, trout, herring, and sardines. Omega-3s improve mental clarity and may decrease the likelihood of depression. Two servings a week is probably sufficient, and farmed fish is probably better than wild fish.

The second prong of care and feeding of the brain is sleep and naps. In our hard-driving culture, we tend to hate downtime and disapprove of sleep and naps. As a result, we are sleeping 45 minutes less per day than a generation

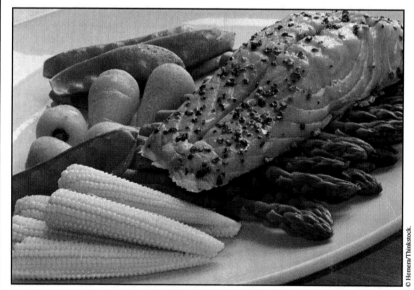

A healthy diet with ample vegetables and fish can improve mental clarity.

ago. But sleep and naps are actually not a waste of time: Sleep-impaired judgment and performance are as disabling as alcohol intoxication. The more people sleep, the better they perform. The top students at any school sleep more than their compatriots.

Consolidation is the fixing of memories that occurs whether we're awake or asleep. Enhancement, which is improving upon what you have learned, occurs during sleep; it's what's called an off-line effect. This all has practical implications: You can improve your learning by scheduling sleep. The initial consolidation of something new takes about 6 hours, so don't take up a new activity within that same framework. Sleep on what you've learned; your brain circuits will be refreshed.

Let's talk about the power of naps. A power nap is nearly as powerful a skill-memory enhancer as a night's sleep. For instance, finger dexterity increases 16% after a nap. Learning facts, words, concepts, and creativity are also improved. But there's a paradox involved in establishing the nap habit: You can't force it. The more you try to force yourself to sleep, the more awake you will be. And naps must be short so as not to interfere with nighttime sleeping. Think of naps as an opportunity for memory consolidation and enhancement, refreshing the brain circuits involved in learning and memory, and an easy way to power down and increase your creative powers.

**The more people sleep, the better they perform.**

The third prong in care and feeding is exercise. The benefits of exercise include increased blood flow and new capillaries around neurons, increased production of new neurons and more interconnections between neurons, and the protection of dopamine neurons from neurotoxins. Exercise also leads to elevations in nerve growth factor and preferentially enhances prefrontal executive processes. The positive balance in neurotransmitters brought about by exercise can even function just like an antidepressant. And a daily 1-mile walk reduces dementia risk by 50%.

We can optimize brain function by paying attention to what we eat, how well we sleep, and how much we exercise. Look for ways to make fitness fun: Get together with friends and take long walks or play a sport. In the next lecture, we'll see how brain optimization can be fun—we'll talk about creativity and puzzles. ■

## Suggested Reading

Arehart-Treichel, "Obesity Linked to Changes in Cognitive Patterns."

Barberger-Gateau, "Dietary Patterns and Risk of Dementia."

Mahoney and Restak, *The Longevity Strategy.*

Morris, "Association of Vegetable and Fruit Consumption."

## Questions to Consider

1. How do your dietary choices impact your brain function?

2. How do the effects of sleep and naps differ?

# Care and Feeding of the Brain
## Lecture 3—Transcript

Welcome to Lecture 3 on the care and feeding of the brain. We're going to take a three-pronged approach; we're going to talk about diet, sleep, and exercise. Now the aim is caloric restriction and weight control and we're going to use a new view, new way of looking at it. Mainly that obesity is cognitively harmful, we'll talk more about that later in this lecture. Controlling ones weight is a way of improving one's brain, simply put. But how much caloric restriction is really necessary? It turns out that the class of foods chosen is less important than the number of calories eaten. Sixty-five years of animal research shows that the rate of degenerative disease is slowed by caloric restriction. Now what do I mean by caloric restriction? It's simply a balanced reduction of protein, fat, and carbohydrates without reduction of nutrient content. It's been shown that animals that eat 35% fewer calories live 35% longer. They not only live longer, but they're smarter and healthier, and they accumulate less of the amyloid seen in Alzheimer disease. They also cognitively outperform animals on unrestricted diets. For instance the Oregon Health and Science research study showed caloric restriction combined with periodic fasting led to better learning and memory performance and exploration of surroundings.

Now would a severely decreased caloric diet work in us, in humans? A National Institute of Aging study showed that a 25% caloric restriction resulted in a lowering of body temperature and insulin levels. This is also seen in calorically restricted animals, which suggests but doesn't prove that such a diet might work. However there's a key point here, few people would be willing to conform to such a diet. Despite the evidence to suggest that caloric restriction of 800–900 calories/day might have a similar effect in humans, it's not feasible or easy to do. I've polled people. You can do it yourself, look up what you would actually be eating when you take in an 800 calorie diet and you may well decide yourself you wouldn't be doing it. Fortunately, such severe restriction may not be necessary. Keeping calories low enough to prevent obesity may be sufficient. Maintaining proper weight is critically important to brain health.

First, several general comments on diets. Diets usually cluster alongside other life-style factors such as drinking and smoking. Not everybody responds the same way to a same food substance, like caffeine for instance. Some people find it alerting and they feel better, other people get coffee nerves. There's also personal taste: George Walker Bush, for instance, use to joke about broccoli, he hated it. An optimal diet for you, while taking these factors into account, should aim at reducing obesity and keeping your weight under control.

Let's explore the harmful cognitive effects of obesity that I mentioned earlier. Animal research shows that diets high in saturated fats lead to underperformance on tests of memory. It also takes longer in tests of reinforcing rewards i.e. pressing a button to get food, it takes longer for an animal to do that. Similar effects are likely in humans—reduction in fats and "empty calories" will improve memory and brain function in general. This has huge implications for a nation like ours with a penchant for fast foods; two-thirds of us are overweight and 30% of us are downright obese. Research suggests high cholesterol and obesity are risk factors for Alzheimer's. Now the new insight is that addiction and obesity are linked together. High-fat high-calorie diets decrease the responsiveness of the brain's pleasure centers. Changes in brain chemistry occur involving dopamine and opioids. This leads to compulsive eating patterns. Obesity and addiction may result from similar maladaptations in the brain's reward systems. Now what's the mechanism for food addiction? Eating is associated with the release of dopamine, and the more dopamine released the greater the degree of pleasure. People with fewer dopamine receptors tend to take in more food to experience pleasure, and they need more food. They are like an addict who needs more and more drug to experience pleasure. The mechanism that we know from animal research that the dopamine receptors decrease in the reward circuitry of the obese and compulsive eating behavior then follows.

So the bottom line is eliminating obesity and doing it without too much effort isn't always easy, but it is worth the effort because of obesity's effects on the brain. You start with "Primum non nocere" which is latin for "first do no harm." Start by eliminating from your diet those foods that can be proven to cause harm. First eliminate trans fats, now these are fats that are formed when liquid oils are transformed into solid fats by adding hydrogen to vegetable oil. Here's a brief history of trans fats: They were introduced to prolong the shelf life in crackers, and cookies, and snack foods. When eaten hydrogenated fats clog arteries in the brain and heart leading to cognitive decline, and memory is especially effected. The stiffer and harder the fat—varying with degree of hydrogenation—the more clogging of blood vessels: like grease on the drain in the kitchen sink. So avoid "hydrogenated" or "partially hydrogenated" foods. And fast foods are the worst: fried chicken, fried fish, biscuits, french fries, potato chips, doughnuts, muffins, things like that. Substitute fruits, vegetables, chicken, whole-grain breads, green leafy vegetables best since they're high vitamin E. Also eat a lot of antioxidants which are chemicals that interrupt oxidation. Think of the rusting of steel beams in a building it's also like plastic degradation. We love plastics because they are so malleable and flexible, they can be molded into any shape that we'd like. Plastics are composed of polymers, which are long chain-like carbon-based molecules, over time oxygen breaks down these bonds through a process called autocatalytic decay, which is a release of chemicals that attack and break down the polymer chains. The end result and end product is acetic acid, which is a vinegar-like substance in terms of its smell.

A similar breakdown process occurs in the body caused by free radical, which are molecular fragments with one unpaired electron and they're rendered unstable. These unstable fragments attract electrons from body tissues such as cell membranes and the structural components of the cell's interior. The membranes or structural components are destroyed by the electron loss and DNA is even eventually attacked. This free radical damage to DNA is partially responsible for aging. Since we can't be sealed in an oxygen-free atmosphere like plastics, we have to take a different approach: Use antioxidants in fruits and vegetables to prolong and protect against free radical damage. The protective effect on brain is dramatic. One study showed that older persons eating more than 2 vegetable servings a day performed as well on cognitive tests as people 5 years younger—this held up over a 6 year follow up. Fruits haven't shown to be quite as effective, but 3 times weekly fruits with vegetables may reduce risk of Alzheimer's disease.

Another important food source: omega-3 unsaturated fatty acids. They're found in oily fish like mackerel, salmon, trout, herring, and sardines. And the greater the intake the more the benefit. Two servings a week probably is sufficient for a person, you don't have to take any more than that. This is the first indication of the benefits of oily fish were seen by psychiatrists. They noted that people living in Japan, Taiwan were 60% less likely to be depressed compared to people in US, where at that time fish was not a staple food. The greater the intake of omega-3s, the lower the rate of depression. It also helped people with the "blues." If the intake of omega-3s increased, depression and/or low mood improved. Today psychiatrists are following up on that and they prescribe omega-3s as antidepressants. It's better that you get these incidentally from fish rather than supplements: lean high-quality protein, vitamins, and minerals like selenium are in fish but they're not found usually in supplements. Two serving of 3 ounces a week is probably enough, and farmed fish is probably better than wild fish because wild fish are leaner with less body fat.

Omegas improve mental clarity. Clinical trial data showed that Alzheimer's improved in early stages by switching to a fish diet. The effect was perhaps due to anti-inflammatory effects interfering with early stages of amyloid formation. You can combine all of this good advice into one diet called the Mediterranean diet consisting of vegetables, fruits, legumes, cereals, olive oil, and fish. Now this is low on meat and dairy products, but it does allow moderate amounts of red wine, in fact they're encouraged.

The second prong of care and feeding is sleep and naps. Sleep and naps are really not a waste of time. In our hard driving culture we sort of hate downtime and therefore sleep and naps are not approved of. As a result we are sleeping 45 minutes less than a generation ago. Sleep impaired judgment and performance are as disabling as alcohol intoxication. When I was in medical school we were kept up for sometimes 36 hours at a time. We couldn't perform our best under those circumstances. In fact the more a person can sleep the better they perform. The top students for instance at any school, sleep more not less than their compatriots.

How much sleep do we need and why? Now the brain doesn't turn off during sleep. Think of the tomato which is storing energy during the day due to photosynthesis and at night using that stored energy for growth. The human brain is sort of like that It takes in information by day and stores it by changing the structure of synapses. Distinctive activity patterns comprising four patterns: REM (or dream sleep) and non-REM. During REM sleep the structural changes are made that I mentioned. Many of the same synapses are used as when we are awake. Dreams involve current concerns, if you think about it it's not a Freudian thing where we think about things that are in the past, most of our dreams are about current concepts since these are the synapses that have been used recently. A Tetris experiment for instance showed that dreams of falling shapes occur to people who have been using Tetris and playing this on a regular basis. During sleep the brain plays same patterns of activity involved in learning and memory during the day. The more learned during the day the greater the replay that night. The point is that the more learned, the greater the need for sleep that night, as I mentioned earlier about good students. Video game players improve according to the strength of hippocampal activation during the night, during their sleep. Consolidation of the information is needed for learning.

Consolidation is fixing memories that occurs whether we're awake or asleep. Enhancement, which is improving upon what you have learned, occurs during sleep: it's what's called an "off line" effect. This all has practical implications; you can improve your learning by scheduling sleep. Let's take tennis as an example. We've all played tennis and after we've played a while we get the "over practice" effect: instead of getting better we get worse. The best thing to do is to stop and return after a night's sleep. The over-practice effect is the result of fatigue of the relevant neurons and circuits. You can combat this by refreshing the circuits by sleep; that way both consolidation and enhancement are both improved. The initial consolidation of something new takes about 6 hours. Don't take up new activity within that same framework; sleep on what you've learned. Your brain circuits will be refreshed. This prevents the interference effect so you don't take a tennis lesson within 6 hours of a golf lesson. The bottom line is here that the 6 hour consolidation rule must be followed. Get in a good night's sleep between sessions whenever possible.

Let's talk about the enemy of sleep: Insomnia. It's a common problem, 43 million sleeping pills are prescribed every year. Here's the definition: Taking more than an hour to fall asleep; wakefulness for over half-an-hour during the night; failure to feel refreshed and rested upon awakening. So what's going on in the insomniac's brain? PET scans show activity in the arousal circuits; this prevents restorative sleep leading to daytime difficulties in learning, memory, concentration, and mood. Sleep deprived rats for instance in the water maze take longer to find the platform when reintroduced to it when learning. They're put in this maze and they can't find the platform if they haven't had a good bit of sleep. test: Sleep fragmentation affects their hippocampus as stress hormones build up and affect circuits for new memories. Insomnia decreases efficiency and you can't perform at your best.

There's also a new concept between depression and insomnia. We use to think that people had sleep problems because they were depressed. Depression may be caused by sleep problems rather than vice versa as traditionally thought. Think back to your last sleepless night. Chances are you weren't lying there thinking about how wonderful the world was, but you were worrying and fretful and you were having personal doomsday scenarios. You were awake not because of worry but you were worrying because you were awake. Take the necessary steps to resolve insomnia. First of all follow methods of sleep hygiene—no stimulants, try to relax, don't review the next day's plans, put your blackberry away, and don't exercise. Next, seek professional help to rule out treatable condition such as obstructive sleep apnea. And finally you may need a short course of sleeping pills that would likely work as long as they largely preserve normal sleep architecture. So a summary of the harmful effects of insomnia are that memory consolidation fails to occur, hippocampal function is interfered with, and the heightened arousal circuits prevent restorative sleep. As a result there are daytime problems in learning, memory, and concentration.

Now let's talk about the power of naps for a second. A power nap is nearly as useful a skill memory enhancer as a night's sleep. Finger dexterity for instance increases 16% after a nap. Learning facts, words, concepts and creativity improved according to the research of Dr. K. Anders Ericsson. Naps also increase off-line learning nearly as much as a whole night's sleep. They increase "sleep spindles," those are the brief bursts of electrical activity seen in regions of new memory formation. But there's a paradox involved in establishing the nap habit: You can't force it. The more you try to force yourself to sleep, the more awake you be. Naps must be short so as not to interfere with night time sleeping. Let me tell you how I established my nap habit. I would set aside 20 minutes in the afternoon just to relax, I tried to get away from forcing anything, and saying I'm just going to relax. I would have my office manager call me after 20 minutes. I would lay there and the first several weeks I didn't fall asleep but then after a while the brain learned that this is the time to take this short nap and this is the time to do this. Now I can do this in almost any time. You can do the same thing, just try it don't force it. Think of naps as an opportunity for memory consolidation and enhancement, refreshing the brain circuits involved in learning and memory, and an easy way to power down and increase your creative powers.

Let's talk about the third prong in care and feeding, which is exercise. There's a generational element here. I'm, for instance, a member of a generation that made firm distinctions between the mental and the physical. As a student, you were either a good student or an athlete. It's very rare that the two of them were combined. Now that has changed, thanks to people like Bill Bradley and Sebastian Coe, the long-distance runner and British MP. It's all because the brain has similar needs to other organs, and we now recognize that. It's not in splendid isolation, it needs glucose, and oxygen, and other nutrients. Now the benefits of exercise included increased blood flow and new capillaries around neurons, increased production of new neurons and more interconnections between neurons, the protection of dopamine neurons from neurotoxins in environment. Exercise also leads to elevations in nerve growth factors; elevations are there when you exercise. Exercise also affects prefrontal executive control processes they're preferentially enhanced. Also brings about a positive balance in neurotransmitters just like antidepressants. In fact a daily 1 mile walk reduces dementia risk by 50%.

Older adults with a history of exercise have better-preserved brains than those who have not exercised of those of the same age according to Arthur Kramer, who's done a lot of research on this. The frontal, parietal, and occipital lobes are most influenced. The frontal and prefrontal lobes focus our attention on what we're thinking about, the parietal and temporal lobes concentrate on what we're doing. This combo results in enhanced memory and focus. As Kramer puts it, "the largest gains involve the executive control processes,... These are the processes that show substantial age-related decline." There are also the processes that distinguish older from younger workers. So here's an important point: a short time frame is sufficient to establish improvement. Just 6 months of regular exercise increases brain volume thus a decreasing volume with aging is really not normal. We thought about that as a normal process for while as a normal process, it really isn't. Just 3 walks of 45 minutes a week is enough to reduce likelihood of dementia by 50%.

Important point: The brain's chemical messenger system is changed by exercise. The same neurotransmitters that are affected with antidepressants, psychiatrists now recommend combining meds and exercise. Exercise lessens chances of Alzheimer's, as I mentioned a mile a day of walking can cut the incidence by 50%. There are also single neuron effects. There are increased neurons in hippocampus. There's greater facility in spatial memory mazes, getting around these mazes. There's an increase in brain-derived neurotrophic factor and other neurotransmitters. In fact there's a positive changes noted in the chemical messenger systems along with an anti-depressant effect. These results were confirmed by a more recent study published in *Neurology*, which is the journal of the American Academy of Neurology, this was done by Kirk Erickson of the University of Pittsburgh. His group reported that walking 6 to 9 miles a week may preserve brain size and consequently stop memory deteriorating in later life.

Nor are the effects of exercise on the brain confined to adults. Two separate studies of 9 and 10 year olds at the Champaign-Urbana campus of the University of Illinois showed that exercise can alter brain structure and improve cognitive abilities. MRIs showed that fitter children scored better on tests of attention. They had significantly larger basal ganglia, which is a key part of the brain that aids in maintaining attention and the executive control needed to coordinate actions and plans. In the second study, this time of complex memory, the hippocampus was found to be larger in the fitter children. In summary, researchers suggest that being fit may enhance neurocognition in young people by increasing the size of the hippocampus and basal ganglia and strengthening the connection between them.

Think of exercise on a continuum model. At one end, exercise is no longer necessary for survival; we don't have any lions we need to escape from, we don't have anything that makes us run on a regular basis to get away from something. On the other end of this continuum are the zealots, these people script their whole lives around compulsive exercising. And I use the word compulsive in a measured way because there's a certain compulsivity about it and they want to have to exercise on a regular basis.

There's also some evidence of a genetic predisposition for exercise. Twin studies show that identical pairs more likely to share exercise patterns. Now these were done from pairs of identical twins that were separated at birth and then studied separately years later. It was found that they had very similar exercise patterns so it suggested that it was all genetic—or at least 60% of it was attributable to genes. There are several variations and several genes related in our response to fatigue, judgments about exercise as being mentally rewarding or not being mentally rewarding, as well as how well the body regulates energy. Now this is something that's under some genetic control, so that one can say that it's all genetics. Any or all of these genes may be contributing here. So here are the implications of the study. Some people may be more drawn to exercise than others but the choice to exercise is still ours to make for the sake of our health.

My personal response to the genetic studies is well, now I don't feel so guilty since I rarely feel the urge to exercise, nor do I particularly enjoy it. But I also recognize that if I had followed a path of only doing what I "felt like" doing I would never have written 20 books about the brain. So even if I'm genetically inclined not to exercise I can find and overcome that limitation. I will just exercise on a regular basis. My personal exercise program consists of about a 35- to 45-minute brisk walking through different parts of Washington DC. So you have to decide for yourself. Do you want to take it to the limit approach to exercise and do as I do and take 3 walks a week for 45 minutes? If you select strenuous exercise instead, I suggest you start with a physical and a stress test. A reading every day about people who suddenly late in life decide they want to do exercising and they will have a heart attack or something like that, it's because they haven't really done this in a measured way. If you haven't exercised up until this time in life and your say beyond 50, you should have a stress test and a physical and then decide what type of program to have. Also decide what benefits are most important to you. Are you after weight loss, improved health, or enhanced cognition?

We can optimize brain function by paying attention to what we eat, how well we sleep, and how much we exercise. If you're like me, you'll look for ways to make fitness fun. Get together with friends and take long walks, I see this in my neighborhood all the time. Ladies and men get together and they walk to Georgetown and various places and they keep busy this way. They make it a communal process. You can try different walking routes and thus combine exercise with learning about your city or town. I use cards outlining 50 walks throughout Washington. Most of them are linked with subways so I can get off the subway and then I can take a 40 or 50 minute walk in a different part of town.

Now the next lecture we're going to show how brain optimization can be fun as we turn from exercise to creativity and puzzles. Thank you.

# Creativity and the Playful Brain
## Lecture 4

William Dement asked his students this riddle: "Consider the letters H, I, J, K, L, M, N, O. Now, this sequence should suggest one word. What is that word?" Some students got it right away. Other ones didn't, and he asked them to dream about it and come in the next day and tell him about their dreams. The students dreamed of hunting sharks, skin diving, being caught in a heavy rain. Does that give you a hint? We're talking about the chemical formula for water: $H_2O$ is the answer, which is the letters H to O in the sequence.

Although everyone agrees about the value of creativity, until recently we knew little about the brain processes underlying it. You may know that the 2 brain hemispheres are specialized: The left is more important for verbal and symbolic processing; the right is important for processing visual-spatial information and is involved with emotional perception and expression. The brain uses the most appropriate hemisphere for a specific task, with assistance from the other hemisphere. For instance, the right hemisphere is not the language hemisphere but can do a little bit of reading. There is an important principle here: You can increase efficiency by activating different brain areas.

Creativity is based on 3 thinking patterns: verbal language, in which unwarranted assumptions can trip us up; music and math, which require the understanding of fundamentals; and visual thinking, which is often the key to creative thinking by envisioning and manipulating information.

Mind wandering (a.k.a. daydreaming) is an everyday power-down state. It's traditionally frowned upon but also very common: 30% of people admit to mind wandering. There's nothing wrong with it: Mind wanderers tend to score high on creativity. When the mind wanders, the brain's executive centers are activated along with a default network. The combination of these 2 networks may explain the link between mind wandering and creativity.

As a practical solution let your mind putter around for a bit so your brain is free to wander productively. But don't overdo mind wandering; it's best in small doses. You need to allow your mind to wander if you want to be creative, but you also need to catch the creative idea. Also important is the contribution of sleep, with or without dreams. Several scientific discoveries have been attributed to ideas that came in dreams.

**We are verbal creatures, and our brains thrive on words.**

Both creativity and divergent thinking involve fluency, which means rapidly producing multiple possible solutions to the problem; elaboration, which means thinking through the details of the problem; flexibility, which means entertaining multiple approaches to the problem simultaneously; and originality, which means coming up with ideas that don't occur to most people.

The goals for divergent thinking are (1) to achieve a spontaneous, random, unorganized, and free-flowing manner of thinking and (2) to loosen the control of the left hemisphere and allow the emergence of less structured, nonverbal material to emerge from the right hemisphere. Some methods for this are brainstorming, mind mapping, and free writing.

Now that we know something about brain geography, let's see how we can use that knowledge to enhance our creativity—and even have some fun in the process. One way to enhance brain function is through creative play. Puzzles, word games, and humor are marked by uncertainty and ambiguity, which test our brains in unaccustomed ways. We tend to resist not having answers to questions that we are asked, which leads to premature closure—reaching a conclusion or accepting an explanation before examining the facts and the logical conclusions flowing from these facts.

I suggest that you embrace ambiguity as a means of enhancing your brain. Puzzles are uniquely appropriate for this. Here's one: What occurs twice in a moment, once every minute, yet never in a billion years? To solve it, forget about analyzing units of time. Think in terms of the words and letters: moment, minute, and a billion years. The answer is the letter "m."

Develop an interest in word games. We are verbal creatures, and our brains thrive on words. As we learn new words, we expand our mental horizons. Word puzzles call on our left hemisphere, which mediates words and language.

Here's a fun word puzzle: Have a friend cut the words from the caption of a cartoon and rearrange them. See if you can restore the punch line by putting the words back in their correct order. Puzzles involving cartoons strengthen the brain's ability to switch points of view and think about things in unusual ways. They also challenge

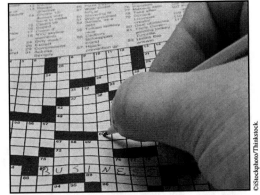

**Challenge yourself with word puzzles; they will enhance your brain function!**

the brain to work with ambiguity and uncertainty. As another word challenge, have someone cut and scramble the frames of a comic strip, and then see if you can rearrange them into their correct order. This exercise tests your puzzle-solving ability, sense of timing, and logic.

So how should we approach solving puzzles? First, just try something! Getting started may be the hardest step. Even a wild guess is fine, because figuring out why the guess doesn't work helps you decide where to focus your efforts. Second, persist! The biggest reason for not solving puzzles is giving up. If you feel you can't persist any longer, then look up the answer. It's OK: Looking at the answer isn't cheating but simply helping your brain learn principles that will be useful in future puzzles. Understand why the answer was correct, and then imagine how you might have gotten the answer yourself. You can also try setting time limits. The brain can almost always work faster if you ask it to.

Puzzles, riddles, and jokes enhance the brain by encouraging reasoning, logic, visual imagination, spatial thinking, working memory, and creativity. Equally important, puzzles, riddles, brainteasers, and jokes are just plain fun! ■

## Brain Teaser

**B**rain teasers can help you enhance concentration, visual thinking, and creativity. Here is one of my favorites.

You are in a room with 3 light switches that turn on 3 light bulbs in another room. You can turn on only 2 of the switches, and you're allowed only 1 trip into the room to check which 2 light bulbs are on. How do you decide which switch turns on which bulb?

There is an unwarranted assumption here—a premature closure. The terms "light bulb," "lights," and "turn on" suggest a visual approach, but think about what other senses might be even more helpful in solving the puzzle. Touch, the most primitive sense, will actually provide the solution.

Have you come to the solution yet? Turn 2 switches on for 10 or more minutes. Turn 1 of them off, and then go into the other room. The bulb that is still lit is controlled by the switch you left on. Now touch the other 2 bulbs. The switch you turned off controls the one that is warm. The third switch controls the other light bulb.

## Suggested Reading

Chatfield, *Fun Inc.*

Edelman and Tononi, *A Universe of Consciousness*.

# Creativity and the Playful Brain
## Lecture 4—Transcript

Welcome to Lecture 4 on creativity and puzzles. In this lecture we're going to talk about what we know about creativity and the brain. Although everyone agrees about the value of creativity, until recently we knew little about how the brain processes it, and what processes are underlying it. Different brain areas are specialized for different functions. Listening to my voice, for instance involves the temporal lobes; watching me the occipital lobes; thinking about lecture points, you use your frontal lobes; and your emotional response to my words involve the right hemisphere and the limbic system.

You may have heard that the two hemispheres are specialized. The left is more important for verbal and symbolic processing. It is the main language center for reading, writing, speaking, and calculation. It also analyzes the right visual field and controls the right hand. Now the right hemisphere is important for processing visual-spatial information such as reading a map or driving in unfamiliar surroundings. It's also involved with emotional perception and expression. It gives the emotional coloring of language, for instance sarcasm. The way we say something like "he's a real brain" being sarcastic, as opposed to "he's a real brain." It also analyzes the left visual field and helps control of the left hand.

The independent operation of the hemispheres was first demonstrated years ago in patients whose corpus callosum had been severed as a treatment for epilepsy. The corpus callosum connects the two hemispheres. But the difference in right and left hemispheric styles has been exaggerated in normals. Each of us has a unique cognitive style that blends the functions of both the left and the right hemisphere.

Brain uses the most appropriate hemisphere for a specific task, with assistance from other hemisphere. For instance the right hemisphere is not the language hemisphere but it can do a little bit of reading. So we have an important principle here: You can increase efficiency by activating different rather than similar brain areas. For instance when you're on the telephone and someone brings you a note, it's a lot easier than when they just come up to you talk to you while you're on that phone. This avoids the interference effect, where the hemisphere functions interfere with each other if activated together.

It's best therefore to arrange things so that you aren't calling on the same brain areas at the same time lest they interfere with each other's performance. For instance, when driving don't try to read road signs while engaging in a spirited conversation. Instead use a GPS which would not interfere as much because you're simply look at it. Now that we know something about brain geography, let's see how we can use that knowledge to enhance our creativity and even have some fun in the process.

Here's our first exercise: Add one mark or symbol to the above Roman numeral (IX) and change it to the number 6. Since IX is a Roman numeral you may be predisposed to think in Roman numerals. Instead, think in terms of other symbols, letters, or numbers. So what symbol, letter, or number would change the Roman numeral IX to the number 6? Well, it'd be the letter "S" of course. The answer is to add the letter "S" to produce SIX. So that's "S" plus the Roman numeral IX. The riddle was solved either by an immediate grasp of the situation—you saw it right away and you had the correct resolution—or you kind of reasoned your way around it or you examined assumptions and got rid of this assumption that it had to be a Roman numeral.

Creativity is often marked by sudden insights—the ah experience, which is a nearly instantaneous insightful resolution of insight that is associated with a sudden burst of activity in the right anterior temporal area, which provides proof that creativity is brain-related. Creativity based on 3 thinking patterns: the verbal language, in which unwarranted assumptions can trip us up—as happened with the IX-six riddle I gave you a moment ago. The second is music and math. Now this of course requires the understanding of fundamentals—we have to know something about math, we have to know something about music. It's dependent on specialized training. The third thinking pattern is visual thinking. Now this is often the key to creative thinking by envisioning and manipulating information.

Now let's look at what is happening in the brain when you come up with a creative solution to a problem. First there's increased involvement of the right hemisphere, especially the temporal lobe. Second there's an increased use of the frontal lobes which are critical for divergent thinking and the coactivation of widespread neuronal circuits. Third is a change in the neurotransmitter system, a modulation of the influence of norepinephrine and the achievement of what we call a power down state, such as rest, relaxation, sleep, especially dream sleep.

Bernard Berenson, the art historian said, "real ideas came to me while relaxed and brooding, meditative, passive way. Then the unexpected happens. An illumination, a combination of words, a revelation for which I had made no conscious preparation." We are talking here of mind wandering, aka daydreaming. That's an everyday power down state. Of course it's traditionally frowned upon but it's also very common: 30% of people admit to "mind wandering. Do you? If so, there's nothing wrong with it. It functions as an escape from boredom for one thing. James Thurber's story "The Secret Life of Walter Mitty" featured a middle-aged man who escaped from boredom by daydreams of himself as a military officer, a brilliant doctor, a heroic bomber. "Mind wanderers" incidentally, score high on creativity. When the mind wanders the brain's executive centers are activated along with a default network. The combination of these 2 networks may explain the link between mind wandering and creativity.

As a practical solution let your mind "putter around" for a bit so your brain is free to wander productively. But don't overdo mind wandering, it's best in small doses: According to Jonathan Schooler a researcher on mind wandering, you need to allow your mind to wander if you want to be creative, but you also need to notice that you are mind wandering and catch the creative idea.

Creative insights emerge from power down states as I mentioned a moment ago. Especially important is the contribution of sleep with or without dreams. Let's discuss 3 examples. The first is August Kekule's dream of the benzene ring, the second is Otto Loewi's dream leading to discovery of the neurotransmitter acetylcholine, and the third was an experiment carried out by William Dement.

Now August Kekule was the discoverer of the chemical structure of the benzene ring, with 6 carbon and 6 hydrogen atoms. He had a dream of 2 intertwined snakes biting their own tails. The dream was based on a grand jury testimony during a murder trial many years earlier; he had been asked to give some testimony. Among the deceased belongings was a signet ring fashioned in the shape of 2 intertwined snakes biting each other's tails. His unconscious memory of this, revisited in his dream and gave him the chemical structure, mainly a 6-layered arrangement composed of carbon and hydrogen suspended like charms from a bracelet.

The second example is Otto Loewi. He believed that the slowing of the heart was caused by a chemical rather than just electrical stimulation. He tried several experiments but wasn't able to demonstrate that. On night he had a dream about how to do it and he woke up and went to the lab. He set up 2 frog hearts and stimulated the vagus nerve of the first heart and then drew off some of that fluid surrounding the heart. He added that fluid to the fluid surrounding the heart of the second frog: That heart too slowed down. We now know that acetylcholine was the chemical released by the nerve cell stimulation of the first frog's heart, and that caused the slowing of the second frog's heart when it was applied to that heart.

In the third example, William Dement, the sleep researcher, asked his students this riddle: "Consider the letters H, I, J, K, L, M, N, O. Now this sequence should suggest one word. What is that word?" Some students got it right away. Other ones didn't, and he asked them to dream about it and come in the next day and tell him about their dreams. The students dreamed of hunting sharks, skin diving, being caught in a heavy rain. Does that give you a hint? We're talking about the chemical formula for water: $H_2O$ is the answer, which is the letters H to O in the sequence.

Now 4 steps can be used to increase creativity. One is to focus on the problem until you really understand it. Mentally put your assumptions into words. Make certain you understand what you must do to reach a resolution. Ask yourself, in other words: What other ways can I think about this and envision this problem in different way?

Now both creativity and divergent thinking involve fluency, which is rapidly producing multiple possible solutions to the problem; elaboration, which is thinking through the details of the problem; third is flexibility, which is entertaining multiple approaches to the problem simultaneously; and finally fourth is originality, which is coming up with ideas that don't occur to most people.

Now creativity employs divergent thinking, which is linking up based on associative memory and novel concepts. It involves the recruitment of distributed cell networks which leads to seeing beyond the obvious. It involves filtering and employing an evaluative attitude. In other words the art and science of the possible, you're not thinking of things that are totally impossible they've got to be reasonable. Third, is the use of a modular versus a linear design, thinking in terms of a mosiac in which something might have to be moved rather than a tightly bound narrative.

The goals for divergent thinking are 1) to achieve a spontaneous, random, unorganized (now not disorganized but unorganized), and free-flowing manner of thinking. Goal 2) is to loosen the control of the left hemisphere and allow the emergence of less structured nonverbal material to emerge from the right hemisphere. The methods for that are like keeping a journal, brainstorming, mind-mapping, and free writing, which means just taking out a journal and start writing as quickly as you can about things that come to mind.

One way to enhance brain function is through creative play. Puzzles, word games, and humor are marked by uncertainty and ambiguity which test our brains in unaccustomed ways. We tend to resist not having answers to questions that are asked us, which leads to premature closure—reaching a conclusion or accepting an explanation before examining the facts and the logical conclusions flowing from these facts. In fact all of us jump to premature and erroneous conclusions. Here is an example: Let me introduce you to Stan. Stan tends to be shy and likes to keep to himself. His apartment is always neat and tidy; typical of his need for order, structure, and attention to detail. Now let me ask you this question on Stan. Based on that description, is Stan more likely to be librarian or a farmer?

Many people would select librarian despite several important considerations. Statistically there are many more farmers than librarians. Words like "shy,:

"neat," and "tidy" activate stereotypes about librarians. As a result we may be less likely to associate these adjectives with farmers than librarians. In our desire for a quick answer and the resolution of ambiguity and uncertainty, we trust in stereotypes. We ignore statistics (such as the base rate that there are more farmers than there are librarians). In fact, Stan's description fits the character only of a librarian written for a movie screen writer unacquainted with many librarians. What's called for in deciding about Stan's occupation was the willingness to avoid premature closure and examine the data.

Let me give you another example. Champagne will keep its fizz overnight if a spoon is suspended in the neck of the bottle and the spoon does not touch the liquid; why is this? That was a question written to the "Last Word" column of the *New Scientist*. To the editors the proposal seemed preposterous and unreasonable. But in the interest of not appearing narrow minded they decided to test it. It worked for 12 hours with even some fizz after 24 hours. Now was this a mysterious insight about spoons and champagne? Well the editors tried a second experiment and asked volunteers to blind taste champagne left overnight with and without a spoon. They found that the spoon had no effect. An incorrect assumption was at work here. That is that champagne quickly goes flat if not corked. Actually it takes about 96 hours before it goes completely flat. You can try it yourself, you can use a bottle of cheap champagne, of course. The bottom line is there is no unexpected "longevity" overnight and thus the spoon had nothing to do with the findings.

We have to train our brain to break through its tendency to leap to premature closure based on seemingly reasonable but incorrect assumptions. A suspension of premature assumptions and judgments is also required for the successful solving of puzzles. Puzzle creators like Scott Kim and David Book ponder for weeks a puzzle's possible solution. They actively resist premature closure. Let's explore how we might do the same.

Think back to brain processes involved in solving the librarian-farmer question. We relied on our memory based on past experience about farmers and librarians. We analyzed the question, the description of Stan. We used our verbal reasoning. We used logic, trying to make sure everything logically followed. And of course we had to keep moving it around in what we call working memory, so we could remember all the components. We also had to have a critical analysis to identify stereotypes, because stereotypes are what threw us off.

In this lecture I am suggesting that you embrace ambiguity as a means of enhancing your brain. Puzzles are uniquely appropriate for this. Try this puzzle: Rearrange the letters in the 2 words NEW DOOR to make 1 word. Before rearranging the letters consider exactly what I requested you to do, now simply do it. You're probably thinking of ways to re-arrange the letters to come up with a novel word. You're probably rapidly going through all of the various possibilities either alphabetically or just guessing. In fact the answer is easy. In fact I've already told it to you. NEW DOOR becomes ONE WORD.

The brain thrives on thinking of things in different ways. Puzzles are prominent and preeminent ways to do this. Here's another one: What occurs twice in a moment, once every minute, yet never in a billion years? To solve it forget about analyzing units of time. Think in terms of the words and letters: moment, minute, and a billion years. The answer is the letter "m."

Puzzles can be divided into 2 types. Those solved by planning, deciding, evaluating, in other words those operations of the frontal lobes. And second those solved by sudden insight, the "Eureka" moment when the answer comes to us in a flash. That involves the anterior temporal lobes, which fire 1/3 of a second before insight. So brain activation actually precedes conscious insight into the answer of the puzzle. So here's a question for you: who solved the puzzle?

Here is another puzzle: At opposite ends are my mouth and my head. I run for miles without leaving my bed. What am I? The sentences are paradoxical: mouth and head at opposite ends? The words must have several meanings; keep thinking about it. "Keep your unconscious riddle-solving machinery on the job" as David Book puts it. Think again. What's the answer? We're talking about a river.

Develop an interest in word games. We are verbal creatures and our brain thrives on words. As we learn new words we expand our mental horizons. We can add extra benefit by playing with words. The book I wrote with

Scott Kim, *The Playful Brain*, uses puzzles to stimulate and optimize brain function. Word puzzles call on our left hemisphere, which mediates words and language. Word puzzles stimulate the language areas in novel ways. We must come up with new and creative arrangements of words. Cross-word puzzles are especially effective at making us think of words in uncommon ways.

As an example of a fun word puzzle have a friend cut the words from the caption of a cartoon and rearrange them. See if you can restore the punch line by putting the words back in their correct order. Here are 3 examples taken from a single issue of *The New Yorker*. so when you encounter a cartoon look, carefully at it and think about what is represented before reading the caption. *The New Yorker* routinely provides cartoons without captions and challenges the readers to provide the caption. Puzzles involving cartoons strengthen the brain's ability to switch points of view and think about things in unusual ways. They also challenge the brain to work with ambiguity and uncertainty.

As another word challenge have someone cut and scramble the frames of comic strip and then see if you can rearrange them into their correct order. This exercise tests your puzzle solving ability, your sense of timing, and logic. After you've mastered the single puzzles, mix 2 or 3 of them together. This comic rearrangement exercise is similar to the basic skills we use when we make plans, tell stories, and anticipate the likely consequence of certain actions. This is primarily a frontal lobe exercise involving timing, sequencing, organization, and executive control. This is similar to the skills needed for sticking to budgets, planning a party, telling a story, or a joke.

So how do we solve puzzles? Here are several of the approaches that Scott Kim suggests in our book, *The Playful Brain*. First, try something. Just getting started may be the hardest step. Even a wild guess is fine because figuring out why the guess doesn't work helps you decide where to focus your efforts. Second, persist! The biggest reason for not solving puzzles is giving up. If you feel you can't persist any longer then look up the answer. Incidentally looking at the answer isn't cheating but simply helping your brain learn principles that will be useful in future puzzles. Understand why the answer was correct and then imagine how you might have gotten the answer yourself.

Now, how to understand and solve form puzzles: I've always had trouble with form puzzles. These are puzzles where you have pieces that are together, like in this box, I can take them out and try to rearrange them. Not so easy actually. Once you have experience with it, such puzzles almost entirely involve the right hemisphere. Putting things into words, which come more naturally to me, doesn't help and in fact it often hinders. How to solve such a puzzle? With the puzzle in place I use a digital camera to take a picture after I remove one piece at a time. Later if I get stuck when I'm working the puzzle, I look at the pictures in reverse order. I am now better at solving such puzzles. This is a good example of Scott Kim's point that we aren't cheating when we look up an answer as long as it helps us organize ourselves and our brain. It is also an example of the use of technology to enhance brain function.

Other suggestions are to set time limits. The brain responds best with a set time limit. The brain can almost always work faster if you ask it to. Now this is the opposite to multitasking; you're doing only one thing but you are doing it faster. We're talking here about brain programming, which is setting a performance goal for the brain and then allowing the brain to fulfill that goal. For instance, I have a habit trying to write between 500 and 1000 words a day. I don't always do it but I prominently display the time available for me to finish that session.

Here's another idea: Use brain teasers to enhance concentration, visual thinking, and creativity. Here is one of my favorites: You are in a room with 3 light switches that turn on 3 light bulbs in another room. You can turn on only 2 of the switches and you're allowed only 1 trip into the room to check which 2 light bulbs are on. How do you decide which switch turns on which bulb? Let's say it one more time: You are in a room with 3 light switches that turn on 3 light bulbs in another room. You can turn on only 2 of the switches and you're allowed only 1 trip into the room to check which 2 light bulbs are on. How do you decide which switch turns on which bulb?

There is an unwarranted assumption here, a premature closure. Light bulb, lights, and turn on suggest a visual approach but think about what other senses might be even more helpful in solving the puzzle? Think of touch, the most primitive sense, actually it will provides the solution. Have you come to the solution yet? Turn 2 switches on for 10 or more minutes. Turn one of them off go into the other room. The bulb that is still lit is controlled by the switch you left on. Now touch the other 2 bulbs. The switch you turned off controls the warm one. The third switch controls the other light bulb.

A puzzle is like a koan, keep thinking about it, mull it over in your mind until it becomes as familiar as the feel of a favorite stone. And forget about it for a while, return to it at odd moments, think of it before going to bed and you may dream about it as with the William Dement dream puzzle. Let's try a puzzle from David Book's *Problems for Puzzlebusters*. From this diagram of 8 quarters laid out in the shape of an L, change the arrangement so that there are 5 quarters in each leg of the L." Now horizontal re-arrangements don't work. You have to think vertically instead of horizontal. The answers is to place one of the quarters from the long arm of the L and place it on top of the quarter in the corner.

Why do puzzles? The strengthen your capacity to concentrate and mull over problems, question initial assumptions, restate and reframe problems, you can shift your mental perspectives—in fact you have to, you can integrate brain function by uniting the activity of the right and left hemispheres. And by doing all of these previous things that I've mentioned you can achieve creative solutions.

Approaches to puzzles involve think of the words in unaccustomed ways. What associations are aroused? What do the objects in the puzzle have in common? Where do you find them? Do they have any parts in common? How can I reorient my thinking?

Humor is also important here because jokes require a similar reorientation. For instance a gymnast goes to the instructor and says, "Can you teach me to do splits?" The instructor says, "I think so. How flexible are you?" The gymnast says, "I can come any day but Wednesday." This is an example of the incongruity- resolution theory. While the set up elicits one line of thinking, the punch line hits us with a different way of thinking.

The frontal lobe plays a active role in the flexible thinking required to get a joke. Frontal lobe damage destroys that flexibility and the person become humorless and literal. As when the doctor says to the patient, "What brought you to the hospital today?" The patient says, "The ambulance." Now sometimes this literalness can be used as the basis for a joke as with the humor of Steven Wright. Here are 2 examples: "Everywhere is walking distance, if you have the time" Secondly, "I saw a bank that said '24 hours banking.' I don't have that much time."

The prefrontal cortex picks up on the incongruity and sends signals to the supplementary area and the nucleus accumbens leading to delighted surprise accompanied by laughter. In depressed people frontal lobe interactions with those structures are decreased. As a result humor is regained only with treatment, which can help. Humor can be used therapeutically: It increases arousal levels, skin conductance, and most important makes the depressed person laugh. The bottom line: Puzzles, riddles, and jokes enhance the brain by encouraging reasoning, logic, visual imagination, spatial thinking, working memory, and creativity. Equally important puzzles, riddles, brainteasers, and jokes are just plain fun!

In later lectures we'll be talking a lot about memory. There's the memory-imagination link. A poor memory function is linked with impoverished imagination. This a new insight incidentally. Similar networks activated by remembering and imagining. We'll learn how to use memory exercises to foster imagination and vice versa. Thus as you improve your memory, your creativity should improve as well, along with concentration, sequencing, facility with numbers, and auditory and visual short-term memory. But before we dive into our memory exercises, we need to learn something about how to focus our attention, which is the basis of improving memory. That's the subject of our next lecture. Thank you.

# Focusing Your Attention
## Lecture 5

> The brain really thrives on getting information and paying attention.
> ... The arts, sports, and everyday living all provide opportunities to
> strengthen attention.

A ttention—also referred to as focus or concentration—must be rock solid to marshal the effort needed to improve your brain's performance. Attention in the mental sphere is akin to endurance in the physical sphere. Like an athlete, you can learn to focus your mental energies, but to do that you must successfully manage challenging factors in our culture: distraction and multitasking.

To be fully attentive, first of all, we have to be awake. This is a fairly commonsense idea; if we're asleep, we're not attending to anything. When we're awake, our attention depends on the degree of wakefulness—if we're drowsy, day dreaming, or stressed, we have decreased focus and attention. We have to be in the narrow continuum where we have highly focused attention; then we'll be able to look at something and get all the details about it.

Let's talk about inattention. As a rule, we don't realize that we're being inattentive. You can think of it as a psychic blind spot. Road accidents, for instance, occur as a result of inattentive drivers and/or pedestrians. We think we see more than we do, and that has consequences. Attention failures are especially serious in our current culture, dominated by fast-response technologies. You're sitting there thinking about something, and you fire off an e-mail before paying attention to the consequences. Or you reach for that cell phone while driving on the highway at 70 mph, leading to an accident.

The biggest impediment to sustained attention in our culture is multitasking. First of all, multitasking is a myth: We're actually doing things sequentially, not concurrently. Interference effects with the use of the same channel dictate that I can only listen to so many conversations at one time. However,

I may be able to listen to a conversation and read something simultaneously, because they're not interfering with one another.

The more people multitask, the worse they do. They become more distractible, and they have problems distinguishing relevant from irrelevant information. There's also loss of organization and of the ability to think for oneself. We need to slow down and pay attention to think most efficiently and creatively—in a word, ponder.

Let's talk about the benefits of attention training. It improves concentration, frontal functioning, I.Q., sequencing, context, drive, and executive control. This lecture guide includes short-term memory exercises that you can use to improve your attention. They will help you with math and reading proficiency, and enhanced performance in attention, concentration, sequencing, and auditory and visual short-term memory. They're also linked with I.Q., which of course is the first thing to decrease with aging.

**Multitasking is a myth: We're actually doing things sequentially, not concurrently.**

Music training is also wonderful for attention. Research shows that after 15 months, structural changes occur in brain circuits used for music processing. Enhanced musical ability is related to motor and auditory skills; in some instances, I.Q. increases as well. Athletics are also good for attention. Sports combine all sensory spheres and eventually lead to the development of what is referred to as muscle memory (but is actually brain memory). Concentrate on your areas of weakness. For instance, if you play tennis and have a weak serve, focus on that.

The greatest challenge that we face in our culture may be trying to enrich our powers of attention while accommodating our society's increasing demands for multitasking. We have to do some multitasking, but we don't want to drive away our attentional powers. In the next lecture, we'll talk about something closely related to attention: memory. If you can't attend, then you obviously can't remember. We'll look at how improving your attentional powers can enhance your memory. ∎

## Short-Term Memory Exercises

Here are some techniques to keep in mind for memory exercises:

- Focus—be sure to pay attention.

- Use as many senses as you can.

- Put the information in the form of an image—the more dramatic the better.

**Visual exercise.** Look at a series of pictures rapidly. Then close your eyes and try to describe them. This measures both your attention and your memory.

**Auditory attention exercise.** Try a game called "Clap Your Name." Let's say your name is Richard. Spell it out, R-I-C-H-A-R-D, by slapping your thigh for each of the consonants and clapping your hands for each of the vowels. You will develop your attention to the auditions, the sound of it. For an added challenge, you can do this simultaneously with someone else.

**Sustained and selective attention exercise.** Quickly dictate into a voice recorder a long string of randomly selected letters and numbers. Later on, listen to them and tally only the numbers or only the letters. This works even better if you get someone else to read them for you: You respond by signaling only when you've heard either a letter or a number.

**Divided attention exercise.** Practice attending to 2 tasks at once. For instance, rapidly tap your finger while attending to a news story on the radio.

**Processing speed exercise.** See how quickly you can shuffle a deck of cards and then break the cards into suits and put them in order.

## Suggested Reading

Restak, *Mozart's Brain and the Fighter Pilot.*

———, *Think Smart.*

# Focusing Your Attention
## Lecture 5—Transcript

Welcome back to a lecture on attention. What happens in the brain when we attend? Attention-also referred to as focus and concentration and it must be rock solid in order to marshal the effort needed to improve your brain's performance. Attention in the mental sphere in fact is like endurance in the physical sphere. Like an athlete you can learn to focus your mental energies, but to do that you must successfully manage 2 factors in our current culture: distraction, which is all around us, and multitasking, which we will talk about today.

Now to be fully attentive first of all we have to be awake, which is a fairly common sense idea. If we're asleep we're not attending to anything. When we're awake, it depends on the degree of wakefulness—if we're drowsy, day dreaming, things like that we're not focused and were not attending. If we're overly stressed, and we'll talk about stress in a later lecture, we're also not attending well and we can't learn about what's happening around us. We have to be in a narrow continuum, right in the middle of it. That's where we have highly focused attention, where we're able to look at something and get all the details about it.

Now there's also a thing called covert attention, which we're not going to necessary that we're attending to. It was Hermann von Helmholtz, who was an early physiologist who wrote about this. He did an experiment which showed it. In his laboratory he wrote out some numbers and some figures on a sheet and hung it up at the end of the hall. Then he turned the lights off and turned them on rapidly to see what he could see on the sheet. He didn't see anything but he found that if he actually voluntarily decided ahead of time what part of the sheet he was going to look at, when the light came on he was able to tell what those letters or numbers were. So he was able to direct his attention to a particular part of the visual landscape and at the same time exclude his attention from all the other parts.

Focusing attention has an effect in the brain. You're changing blood flow patterns, in this case to the visual areas of the brain. So when Dr. Helmholtz was looking at this he was actually increasing blood flow to the visual part of the brain. It was highly specific; we learn about the world by turning our attention to certain parts of it. There's also a linkage between intention and attention, just as in Helmholtz's experiment. We decide to do something and then we devote our attention to it. Now that can be used in a magic trick for instance, when a magician, for instance, will distract your attention. He'll say "look at this" and when you do, the actual magic trick is taking place elsewhere, so that you've been tricked. The audience is directed to intentionally focus in on something that's not important to the trick.

Now if you look at this particular image. It shows you that the upper part of the brain the attentional network can control what we're paying our attention to—just like Helmholtz decided to look at a certain part of that screen. However we also have sensory input coming from the various senses. If we're stung by a bee, for instance our attention is directed right there. So it's a dynamism when you think about, between focusing our attention up here, the upper part the frontal areas particularly, and our attention being captured by events happening around us.

The brain effects of attention are enhanced activity in various parts of the brain—the frontal, parietal, the insular cortex, plus an important area called the anterior cingulated. Now these all comprise a vast attentional network. Each has a particular thing that it does: The parietal formulates a dynamic representation. The frontal lobe formulates an action, what's going to be done. And the limbic determines motivation. In this picture you can see all of these different areas shown, so this is the attentional network we just talked about.

If attention is not being paid it can be due to damage in the brain. We'll talk about those first, then we'll talk about normal types of inattention. If you have damage to the right parietal lobe of the brain, which is right up here, then you aren't paying attention to things on the left side—the things that you would see, feel, touch, and bodily integration. For instance a man won't put his arm into the left sleeve of his shirt because of this inattention of his left side. Now it's not just all the right parietal lobe, the opposite parietal lobe is also involved. So right, plus left, as well as the frontal lobe to a lesser extent. Now in this picture you can see what happens in someone who has damage in the right parietal lobe. They're asked to put a dot in the middle of a line and as you can see the line is moved off to the right because they're not attending to the left side. The other thing they're asked is to make crosses out of these figures; you can see it's not done on the left side, it's only done on the right. There's also a picture of a clock, which someone is asked to draw the face of a clock and they're only able to draw the right side because they've extinguished the left side.

As a rule we don't realize that we're being inattentive. We're talking now, we've moved from people with damaged to normal brains. You can think of it as a psychic blind spot. We have a visual blind spot, that's for the optic nerve that leaves the back of the eye and goes into the brain. There's a psychic blind spot as well, things we don't pay attention to. Road accidents for instance occur as a result of inattentive drivers and/or pedestrians. The military has an interesting exercise in which they will suddenly ask a Marine to close his eyes and give a description of what room they're in, where the windows are, how they would escape, where things might happen. Then they open their eyes and they check it out. This is an example of an attention exercise.

All of us are prone to inattention. There's a famous experiment that illustrates this very nicely. It's called Gorillas in our Midst, by Christopher Chabris and Daniel Simons. If you want to try it for yourself, pause the lecture now and look it up in your favorite search engine. The experiment presents you with a video of 2 basketball teams. There's a team wearing a black jersey and team wearing a white jersey. While each team passes the ball back and forth you're instructed to count the number of passes that the white team makes. Now you know there will be trick, so make sure to pay close attention to those players. And in the experiment while you're counting, something unexpected happens: A gorilla walks across the basketball court directly past the players. Now most people are so focused on the ball they don't notice the gorilla at all. Try the experiment again now that you know the outcome; the gorilla seems obvious now doesn't it?

Christopher Chabris and Daniel Simons say that our picture of reality is inherently incomplete, though, most of the time we think that we don't realize how much we miss. We think we see more than we do, and that has consequences. If we were aware of our limitations we wouldn't text or drive or think of anything else that would cause us to have problems in terms of remembering. Attention failures are especially serious in our current culture, dominated by fast-response technologies. You're sitting thinking about something and you fire off an e-mail before paying attention to the consequences. Or you reach for that cell phone while on the beltway at 70 mph and during that tenth of a second distraction you are involved in a fatal accident. Now if your attention failure is a chronic one you may be suffering form attention deficit hyperactivity disorder (ADHD). Perhaps attention disorder is a consequence of our technologically fast paced society? It may well be and we're going to talk about that a little bit later. In fact, Elias Aboujaoude, the director of Stanford University's Impulse Disorders Clinic, has this to say about our attention spans:

> One reason that ADD is on the rise is that our attention span is similar to our attention span on Facebook. Look at language. People are writing the way they text. Anything complex that takes several paragraphs to develop is information overload. I think it is regressive, not progressive. It is becoming so normalized in our culture, it becomes hard to catch while it's happening.

While keeping in mind our brain's inattentional failures under certain circumstances called "inattentional blindness," let's return to the positive benefits of learning to focus our attention like a laser. There's 3 attentional control systems in the brain we have to think about. The first is the alerting system, which is in the frontal lobe and the parietal areas and used as the neurotransmitter, or messenger, dopamine as the active messenger. Second is the orienting system, which is frontal and temporal, plus the temporoparietal junction, and that uses acetylcholine as the messenger. And third is an executive system also frontal cortex. It also uses dopamine as the messenger.

Now first of all you have to think about the brain as purpose driven. A forest for instance can inspire a poem, a botany lecture, or a scheme for leveling the trees in the interest of development. Each goal is enhanced by attention, focusing on how to modify current status in order to achieve intended goals. There are benefits from enhanced attention: improved frontal functioning, I.Q. improves; sequencing, context, drive, and executive control. We talked about those in the lecture on the frontal lobe. We also have improved conflict resolution by learning what to attend to and what to ignore because we don't want to attend everything in our world, everything around us. That's the definition of hyperactivity attention disorder. We want to actually focus our attention, as we said earlier, like a laser.

We want coordination of scattered networks involving sensation, movement, emotions, and language. Any of those things can be the object of our attention. We can be attending to what we're feeling; I gave the example before of being stung by a bee. We could be attending to our movements, how we're feeling, our emotions, and our language. Interestingly, attention has a calming, focusing effect which you can feel as you try it yourself. It's often described in those with a tiny bit of ADHD.

There are impediments to a sustained attention. You remember the picture we looked at earlier when you went from sleep to alertness? This is an example of what's called the Yerkes-Dodson Law, where there's an optimal level of alertness that you should have to be attentive. Too much or too little and you're not attentive. Second impediment is boredom. Third is emotional blunting or "burn out," after a while we've done things over and over we tend not be attentive and day dream. Next is sensory overload, there are simply too many things coming on at one time. The biggest impediment in our culture to sustained attention is multitasking.

There are arguments pro and con for multitasking, so let's explore in a little bit of depth here. First of all as many people speak of it, multi-tasking is a myth. We're actually doing things sequential not concurrently, we switch from one thing to the other but we're not doing them both at the same time. That's what's called an interference effects with use of same channel, for instance I can only listen to so many conversations at one time because one interferes with the other. Now sometimes OK if you have separate channels, I can listen to a conversation and be reading something because they're not interfering with one another. While talking on the phone I can be reading notes, things like that.

Mental channels can also interfere with physical channels, not many people realize that. Here's an example: You're driving along in your car and you're on your cell phone, which you shouldn't be for reasons which we'll talk about in a moment. You're talking to your architect about doing some work in your house. So now you're using the part of your brain that you're imagining this particular renovation, you're using the same part that you're supposed to be using as you're driving and weaving your way through traffic. There's a bottle neck at the frontal lobe, which interferes with us being able to consider 2 things truly at the same time; it's more that it's sequential. Now this is the example of cerebral geography.

Have you ever noticed that when you're trying to make up your mind about 3 things it's particularly difficult? We're much more comfortable figuring out 2 things. There's a reason for that. Difficulties arise when we have 3 or more, we tend to discard 1 of them. For deciding to go to the beach, the mountains, or NYC we tend to eliminate 1 of them and make our decision between the other. Discard 1 and choose between the other 2. The reason for that is that the brain is binary because medial frontal cortex divides one half into one choice and the other half on the other choice. The medial frontal cortex is part of the brain's motivational system, where rewards are represented. In an experiment matching upper and lower case letters, each side was encoded on one side or the other of the medial frontal cortex. With the introduction of a third letter in this matching test, efficiency dropped precipitously. It was as if each hemisphere was occupied in managing one task and there was nowhere for the management of a third task. Bottom line: Reduce your decision tree to no more than 2 alternatives. Binary multitasking is really about all we can handle because of how our brain is constructed. That's not a weakness, it's just that's the way we are.

Let's talk about the consequences of multitasking. The more people multitask the worse they do. They become more distractible, and they have problems distinguishing relevant from irrelevant information. Also problems with mental file keeping, knowing where to put things in conceptual boxes, knowing exactly where they are and you can access them. There's also loss of organization, they become much disorganized. The inability to think is also important. That's applying sufficient attention and concentration to develop one's own ideas; think for oneself. First ideas often seem to be brilliant, but they're superficial and derivative. Twitter, tweets, and YouTube provide you with other people's ideas. Raw unorganized data. To form associations and connections you need time and the absence of distraction. You need the absence of multi-tasking. So slow down and pay attention in order to think most efficiently and creatively. In a word: ponder.

Depth, clarity, and cohesion of thought take time and focused attention. All 3 are impaired by multitasking. As the novelist and essayist, Jay Griffiths, has written "Skim-talking and skim-reading promote skim-thinking. Thoughts that are summoned at speed are likely to be not the best but simply the first."

I mentioned a moment ago about driving a car and talking on a cell phone, which is deathly not to do because of the interference effect as I described it. Now David Strayer, who actually did this work and showed that talking on a cell phone actually impairs your ability to drive almost as much as you being intoxicated, actually found that there is a very, very small number of people (2.5 %) who we call "supertaskers." These are people who did just doing 2 things as doing 1. He's written about them, he says "There are supertaskers in our midst: rare but intriguing individuals with extraordinary multitasking ability … [in these individuals the] multitasking regions may be different the brain may actually if you want to put it this way organized differently." There's a problem with that finding if you think about. Everyone, all of us, will assume that he or she is among that 2.5%. Everybody is always "above average." I know on examinations and things when I've taught people in large crowds, I've said, "How many people think they're above average in this group?" and everybody's hand goes up. Well that of course creates a problem because if in fact everybody is above average what does the term average really mean?

Let's talk about the benefits of attention training and what it does. At the end of the lecture I'm going to give you ways of focusing your attention and improving it but now let's talk about the benefits of attention training. It improves concentration, performance in tests of general intelligence. Your EEG, your electroencephalogram, shows increases in anterior cingulate activity which correlates with improvements in emotional control. I mentioned a little bit earlier, the anterior cingulate is part of the brain that has to do with emotional control. Working memory exercises correlate strongly with attention enhancement—as I've mentioned working memory, which will be a topic of whole lecture, is basically doing a little bit of juggling in your mind so you're taking things from your memory and you're moving it around.

Inattention, of course, is the most common cause of forgetting. We say why did I forget, we weren't encoding anything. We meet somebody at a party later we worry that we can't remember their name because we weren't really listening. We didn't encode and therefore we can't retrieve. Stress focuses up to a point, but as I mentioned with the Yerkes-Dodson Law, if you get too much stress you can't attend at all. Also attention varies with interest. We all have various things that we're interested in and we are very attentive. Even people with ADHD can perform normally if they're interested in the topic.

Now there are short term memory exercises that I'm going to give you. One of them is called a forward digit span. This is the first of ones that you can use to improve your own attention. I'm going to tell you what it is in just a second, but I'm going to tell you what it can do. It'll help you with math and reading proficiency, enhanced performance in attention, concentration, sequencing and auditory and visual short-term memory. It's also linked with I.Q., which of course is the first thing to decrease with aging. There's different encoding for this as well than there is in general memory.

Let me talk a bit about the memory techniques that we'll use. First is focus, pay attention. Use as many sensory factories as you possibly can. And put the information in the form of an image, the starker the better; the more dramatic the better. Create and learn a system of memory pegs based on your life experience. I'm going to tell you exactly how to do that in a special lecture on how to establish a superpower memory.

Relating attention exercises to teaching, we have things like visual, look at pictures rapidly and then close our eyes and try to describe them, which is a measure of not only our attention but also our memory. We also have auditory, listening and recalling exactly what we've heard. There's a game called "Clap Your Name." Let me describe it to you for auditory attention where you say your name, let's say your name is Richard as mine is, and you take the consonants and you slap your thigh and the vowels you clap your hands. R-I-C-H-A-R-D. You're name may be Maria, so it would be M-A-R-I-A. Now you learn to do that, you get this attention to the auditions, the sound of it. You can play it with someone else, and of course you will be momentarily confused because one will interfere with the other but you're able to do this after some practice.

A proprioceptive attention game is Jenga, which is a game involving a tower of blocks. You remove one at a time carefully, paying great attention to your hand movements, to your spatial movements without collapsing the whole thing. So this is one of proprioceptive attention. You can also do drawing supplemented by verbal description. You say I'm going to make a drawing of something and supplement that with a verbal description. These are attention exercises that you can use.

Improving various components is important, because with attention there's not just one. There's sustained attention, divided attention, selective attention, and processing speed. Let me talk about each of them separately. Sustained and selective attention is something like quickly dictate into a voice recorder a long string of randomly selected letters and numbers. Real quick, and later on listen to them and tally only the numbers or tally only the letters at the end of the list. This works even better if you can get someone else to read it for you. Random letter-number list and you respond by signaling only when you've heard one or the other. Divided attention is attending to 2 tasks at once. It's a little bit like multi-tasking but it's an exercise that you can do. Same period of time, like rapidly tapping your finger while listening and attending to a news story on the radio. Processing speed is another way of attention. Shuffle a deck of cards and break the cards into suits from ace to deuce, how fast can you do this? That's an attentional mechanism.

Music training is really great for attention. Research on music shows that after 15 months structural changes occur in brain circuits used for music processing. Enhanced music is related motor and auditory skills, so the better you get the better motor and auditory skills you have. In some instances I.Q. increased as well. So It's never too late to take up music, in fact I highly recommend that no matter your age. Michael Posner, who's a neurologist who's written quite a bit on the arts on music and the arts says that "music training can change brain circuitry, and in some instances, improve general cognition...The key factor is diligence. Practicing for long periods of time ... and with sustained focus can produce stronger and more efficient attention networks, and these key networks in turn affect cognitive skills more generally."

I gave you the example a few minutes ago of "Clap Your Name," which is a game that strengthens your ability to attend to musical rhythms. You actually converted your name into a musical rhythm. It's an interesting experience as I said to do it yourself, then with someone else, then get a group together. It's almost like a quartet or something, each one is listening to the other musician but they're also playing their particular instrument.

Athletics are also important in attention. It combines all sensory spheres, such as golf, tennis, any team or solitary sport is fine. You eventually develop what they call muscle memory, but that's not muscle memory it's brain memory. The setting up of circuits within the brain, what's sometimes called embodied knowledge. Concentrating on areas of weakness for instance, if you're playing tennis instead of just doing the same thing again and again. Find out is it the weakness of the serve that you want to improve, then you would concentrate on that. Of course there are ego issues, aren't there? Nobody wants to admit that there's something that they're not good at. That's the other side of a professional. Also they can overcome these sorts of ego issues. Also there's habit and repetition compulsion. We tend to do the same thing over and over, because it's comfortable. We've learned how to do it, so why not just hit the same number of golf balls again and again, instead of really focusing on the fact that you need to put some attention on putting.

Improved attention, if I can summarize for a bit, can lead to cognitive enhancement in multiple, multiple areas. You can identify impediments to attention in your own life. Just think what are distractions, what keeps you from focusing? Remember I said earlier there's a certain nice feeling that you get from focusing and really paying attention. The brain really thrives on getting information and paying attention. You can train your ability, which is very important, to pay attention: improvements in sense memory, general memory, and working memory. The arts, sports, and everyday living all provide opportunities to strengthen attention. For example, as you're sitting there now, who is sitting beside you? You know who it is, but what exactly are they wearing? Did you pay any attention to it? What color is her dress? "What type of a neck tie is he wearing? Sometimes we're moving through life and we're not really paying attention. We're missing a lot. The aim is to balance attention improvement with multitasking demands.

In summary, attention and memory are highly interrelated and by enhancing one you enhance the other. Think of attention as a conduit for sharpening other cognitive skills. Here are the practical tips: When you become inattentive and lose focus, it's time to quit what you're doing, perhaps take a nap as we said in care and feeding of the brain. Another practical tip: Discover your own personal attention duration, we all vary in that our work habits and such. Some writers write all day long, other writers can only work 20 minutes at a time, they have to take a break then come back. It varies quite a bit.

Our greatest challenge that we face in our culture that I think is to enrich our powers of attention while accommodating to our society's increasing demands for multitasking. We don't really have a choice about multi-tasking, we have to do a little of it. But we don't really want to drive away our attentional powers. Let me just read from what a friend of mine and novelist, Phyllis Theroux, it's a lovely quote when she states about the powers of attention. Phyllis Theroux says, "Looking back … I see the idea of attention, pure attention, emerging in different forms and guises. Slowing down long enough to pay full attention requires an empty mind. We must clear the decks and be nothing else. This is what goes counter to the culture, which tries to distract and divide our attention so that it never rests on any one thing for any length of time."

In the next lecture, we'll talk about something that's very clearly related to attention, and that's memory. Cause if one can't attend then you can't obviously encode or remember. So the next lecture will be on how improving your attentional powers can enhance your memory. Thank you.

# Enhancing Your Memory
## Lecture 6

**A lot of times we go through life without remembering what we're doing. Have you ever noticed someone looking at a watch and then a second later you ask them, "What time is it?" and they look again? Why would that be? Didn't they just look? Don't they remember exactly what they saw? It's an example of where we are not paying attention to our sensory input.**

With this lecture, we begin to explore the many forms of memory and what you can do to improve your memory. When you think about it, memory is the natural extension of attention and learning. You can't use information that you can't recall—but you can't recall what you haven't attended to. The act of memory facilitates the formation, activation, and retention of circuits that contribute to the brain's optimal functioning. In a way, we are the sum total of the memory we retain. Without memory we wouldn't know who we were.

Memory is controlled by a key region, the hippocampus, which regulates the inward flow of information prior to its distribution to the rest of the brain. Memory forms the basis for personal identity and is also key to thinking. Hippocampal disease is accompanied by disturbances in memory— Alzheimer's disease is a well-known example. Recalling the past and imagining the future are both functions of the hippocampus. To imagine a future event, you have to have some memory of many past events.

The plethora of technology in our modern society means we don't have to remember things. This leads to disuse atrophy—but you can overcome it by deliberate effort to improve your memory. This can stave off Alzheimer's disease, hone your attentional abilities, and link memory with other cognitive processes such as learning and creativity. Some people have great memories—you ask them something, and they're able to tell you the answer and to remember it even months later. Other people have weak memories. The distinguishing feature is retrieval. Memories are best coded and retrieved when linked with an image or an emotion.

There are many types of memory, but here we will concentrate on declarative memory. Declarative memories are consciously accessible memories that are infinite. Vocabulary is a good example; there's no limit to how many words you can learn. A nondeclarative memory, in contrast, is something that really can't be put into words. Knowing how to ride a bicycle or do a double-flip off a diving board are examples of nondeclarative memory. These are things that you have to learn by doing.

**The most important principle for improving your memory is focusing your attention on what you're trying to learn.**

Remember: The most important principle for improving your memory is focusing your attention on what you're trying to learn. You should start with sense memory because that's the brain's initial recording of physical sensations as they impinge on our sense organs. This includes what we see, hear, touch, taste, and smell. Too often, sensation occurs outside of awareness. Here are some exercises that can help you enhance memory via heightening your conscious awareness.

A powerful short-term memory strengthening exercise is called the digit-span exercise. Try it first with auditory recall. Read into a recorder a series of 5-, 6-, 7-, and 8-digit strings. You'll probably want to group them so that all the 5-digit strings are together, the 6-digit strings are together, and so on. Then put them aside for a while and clear your mind. Several hours later, listen to the lists, pause, and then write down as many of the strings as you can recall. Then play the recording to check for accuracy. You can also do this exercise visually by writing the digit lists on a piece of paper. Write a list, turn it face down, look at it quickly, and then try to remember the sequence. The visual and auditory spans focus attention and concentration. A typical adult digit span is between 5 and 7. Start at 5 and build it up through practice.

Why bother to practice and lengthen the digit span, you might ask? Don't be fooled by the apparent simplicity of this exercise; this is a powerful way of improving brain function in multiple areas. The digit span is a predictor of math and reading abilities and of enhanced performance in attention, concentration, sequencing, and auditory and visual short-term memory.

Short-term memory needs to be in active rehearsal in order to be moved to long-term memory. But rehearsal alone isn't sufficient; depth of processing is required. Rote repetition is not as effective as working with the information. Memorization of dates, for instance, is not as effective as writing an essay on what happened on a particular date. Depth of processing increases the web of connections among stored memories.

Repeated testing is also key for long-term memory. Tests should include old as well as new material. Do you remember those ornery professors

## Spices and Sense Memory

Olfaction sensory fibers are the most direct point of sensory input—they connect directly to the brain. Let's sharpen our special senses of taste and smell. Start by taking an array of spices and setting them out on a table. Close your eyes, and identify by smell alone such things as oregano, mint, minced onion, sage, sweet basil, orange, cumin, and black pepper.

Next, take this knowledge and progress to identifying spices in a meal that you are eating. If you're in a restaurant, ask what spices the chef used. When you're making a meal with spices, try not putting the spices in a certain half. Do you taste the difference?

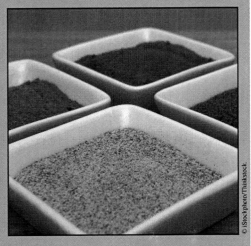

© iStockphoto/Thinkstock.

from college who unexpectedly went back and retested you on things you had already been tested on? Well, it turns out those professors were on to something. Repeated testing is more effective for long-term learning. Why? The neuronal networks are strengthened each time the memory is retrieved. It's similar to physical training: After you build up a muscle or muscle group, you have to keep exercising it to avoid disuse atrophy.

In our next lecture, we'll discuss the most important memory process of all—working memory. ■

## Suggested Reading

Gluck, Mercado, and Meyers, *Learning and Memory.*

Schacter, *The Seven Sins of Memory.*

# Enhancing Your Memory
## Lecture 6—Transcript

Welcome back. Today we will begin the first of 3 lectures exploring the many forms of memory and what you can do to improve your memory. When you think about it, memory is the natural extension of attention and learning that we spoke about last time. We can't use information we can't recall. But you can't recall what you haven't attended to. The act of memory facilitates the formation, and the activation, and retention of circuits that contribute to the brain's optimal functioning. In a way we are the sum total of the memory we retain. Without memory we wouldn't know who we were. Take out a photo album; observe its power to evoke memories that were previously irretrievable. You see things in there you forgot about and suddenly it comes back to you because of this picture. Now the new digital cameras make it possible to date each picture and some even have GPS so that you can get an exact fix on where you were when you took the picture. A diary or a journal can provide similar methods for testing and aiding memory.

But memory is too important to delegate it to our technological tools. Without our memory we truly don't know who we are because we can't bind the past and the present to provide a launching point for creating our future. It's our memory gives our frontal lobes something to work on. We have loses of memory in fictional examples, such as the character in Chris Nolan's Memento. If you remember Leonard Shelby, he suffered a profound memory loss. Now that was fiction, but there are also real life equivalents. There's a famous patient known as H. M., who couldn't form new memories after surgical removal of the hippocampus and parts of anterior temporal lobes on both sides of his brain.

We're going to say a lot about the hippocampus, it's the entry portal for information to be remembered. If hippocampus is damaged we have difficulty forming new memories, as with H. M. Now, H. M., whose real name was Henry Molaison, started having seizures when he was 10 years of age. By age 20 he was completely incapacitated. He couldn't work, couldn't form relationships, lived at home with his mother because at any time he could be felled with one of these horribly sudden total seizures. At age 27, in 1953, he underwent a new operation. Now not the corpus callosum operation that we talked about last time where you split the hemispheres by cutting the corpus callosum and winding up with a split brain perforation. This was a different type of surgery. A finger-sized portion of the anterior temporal lobe was removed containing both hippocampi.

After the operation H. M. seemed to be normal at first hour or so, but then very unusual things were noticed. He could no longer learn and remember new information for more than a few seconds. In fact for a time, people thought maybe he was putting them on. They would come in and introduce themselves, then they'd leave and come back and he wouldn't remember who they were. This is the way it was for his whole life actually. After meeting someone new he couldn't recall meeting them just a few minutes later and had to be reintroduced. It was so bad at one time that after his mother had died, they said please don't tell him that because each time someone mentions it to him he grieves again because he doesn't remember that this occurred. He remembered things clearly that had happened before the operation but he couldn't form new memories of things after the operation. This includes names, events, places—all were forgotten almost immediately. Over the years his face in a mirror surprised him because he only remembered what he looked like as a young man. Every question was new, even if asked moments before.

In 1993 his psychologist played a tape for me—I was doing a book at the time on memory. This was a conversation she had with H. M. He had no memory of what he did early in the day or anybody he had met that day. He wasn't certain of her identity even though she had worked with him for 25 years. When she told him he should know who she was, he kinda got a little bit reticent and he said, "Well, I think you and went to high school together." Now throughout this discussion of the tape I was hearing, he sounded very tentative—he wasn't convinced of her assertions or what she was asking him. What he said he didn't sound like he was very clear about. Finally, with fatigued resignation he admitted that his memory was severely deficient.

H. M. died on December 2, 2008 at the age 82. Since then his brain has been dissected and converted into high resolution digital images. Jacopo Annese, who was doing this, describes it as "a neurological biography that survives in glass and pixels." H. M.'s tragic experience led to the new insight that memory is controlled by a key region, the hippocampus, which regulates the inward flow of information prior to its distribution to the rest of the brain where it becomes long-term memory.

Memory forms the basis for personal identity, as illustrated by H. M. Memory is also key to thinking. "The art of remembering is the art of thinking," as William James put it years ago, one of the foremost psychologists of the 19th and early 20th centuries. Memory involves chemical and structural changes as well. I'm thinking now of the Nobel Prize winning Eric Kandel's work on Aplysia, or the so-called sea slug. When the gill is touched, or poked, the gill tends to retract. The more it's poked, the more this particular reflex comes out. So repetition favors memory consolidation. Now of course that goes all the way up to our own species. Consolidation is favored by repetition, that's why we study. There are also neurotransmitter concentration changes; neurons grow and form new synaptic terminals. We have both biochemical and anatomical changes. New proteins are needed to produce these changes and new connections are made, the synapses. If the repetition of the experience decreased, the number of synapses also decreases. So there's a relation there between the stimulation, the chemistry, and anatomy.

The bottom line is that synapses are not fixed but change with learning. We discussed this in Lecture 3 on plasticity. Memory encoding also involves molecular changes within the neurons. Short-term memories involve more than simply the transmission between one neuron and another, this particular neurotransmitter called glutamate is altered, but also there are interneurons that produce serotonin, which sort of tune the release of the neurotransmitter glutamate. This fine tuning occurs through a series of cascading molecular signals that eventually lead to modification of the cell nucleus of the neuron. You're actually changing the genetics of the neuron through these experiences—another example of epigenetics that we talked about before. If the changes delve right into the neuron, as they do, then you're going to change the whole structure of the neurons in terms of its biology and biological destiny.

Memories are thus the result of an elaborate process involving chemical and genetic signals that result in new synaptic terminals. Eric Kandel talked about this. In fact there's a quote that I'd like to read from him. He said, "short-term memory produces changes in the function of the synapse, strengthening or weakening pre-existing conditions; long-term memory requires anatomical changes." Unlike computer memory, the brain is always in a state of renewal. Memory is also influenced by emotions, which have different valences depending on the situation. If I asked you to remember September 11, it's not just a date it's a specific event which occurred on September 11, 2001. If you're old enough, try to remember where you were and what you were doing when you heard about the death of JFK, John Fitzgerald Kennedy. You see recalling a memory restarts the process of consolidation; it involves emotions as well. Starts again as a short-term memory and then proteins produced for consolidation to for long-term memory. Thus remembering is a creative act that can't be duplicated by a computer. Joseph LeDoux, whose done a lot of research on memory and he has a good quote regarding that. As he puts it, "the brain that does the remembering is not the brain that formed the initial memory. In order for the old memory to make sense in the current brain, the memory has to be updated." It's almost Proustian in a way, the idea that your personality is changing as time goes on because of memory. This has important implications of this new understanding of memory. The Greek philosopher, Heraclitus said you can't enter the same river twice, meaning it's always changing. You also can't remember the same experience exactly alike on different occasions. The you of today, in other words, is different from the you who was present a very short while ago, or who remembered and earlier consolidated a memory. So with this as background let's return to the hippocampus—the starting point for all memories as we have seen with H. M.

Hippocampal disease is always accompanied by disturbances in memory. Alzheimer's disease is probably the most frequently attributed disease that we talk about. Mild hippocampal atrophy also occurs in depression. As depression gets better through antidepressants, you begin to see normalizing of the size of the hippocampus as memory normalizes. I use to a test with patients. I give them 4–5 items to remember like apple, tie, pen, house, car and see if they can repeat them 5 or 10 minutes later. Which is a test of the encoding in the hippocampus. The recollection of the past and imagining the future functioning are also part of the hippocampus. Imagining a future event, you have to have some memory of many times a past events. Both memory and imagination are impaired in Alzheimer's disease, which is the extreme loss of memory and sadly, the loss of self.

Physical applications such as using memory exercises as a means to foster imagination and vice versa are seen in writing schools, for instance. A young aspiring novelist will be asked to go into a restaurant and listen to conversation to get the exact way people talk. He can use that later in a novel and form highly specific images and later write them down. A camera can be used. I use a little 15-second clips. I have a small camera that takes still pictures primarily but it also takes little movies. I'll take a 15-second clip of something and then later I'll look at. Then later try to remember what I saw and use that to try to enrich my memory.

Why not rely entirely on electronic memory aids? The reason is that this would lead to disuse atrophy. In Plato's *Phaedrus*, Socrates refers to the Egyptian god Thamus on the invention of writing, which is really very similar to what we're thinking about now when we talk about memory: "This invention will produce forgetfulness in the minds of those men who learn it, because they will not practice their memory. Their trust in writing, produced by characters which are not part of themselves, will discourage the use of their own memory within them."

Today's disuse atrophy comes from technology: Nothing has to be remembered. But disuse atrophy can be overcome by deliberate efforts to improve your memory. This helps stave off Alzheimer's disease; it hones your attentional abilities; it links memory with other cognitive processes such as learning and creativity. There are good and bad memories as you know. Some people have great memories, you ask them something and they're able to tell you the answer to remember it, and tell it to you months later. Other ones have kind of bad memories. The key is retrieval; retrieval is the distinguishing feature. Memories are best coded and retrieved when linked with an image or an emotion—the basis for memory techniques that we will cover in Lecture 12.

There are many types of memory but here we will concentrate on declarative memory. They are consciously accessible memories and they're also infinite. Vocabulary is a good example; there's no limit to as many words you can learn. That's an example of declarative memory. A nondeclarative memory is something that really can't be put into words. You riding a bicycle, for instance, is a nondeclarative memory. Doing a double-flip off a diving board is another example. You can't really tell people how to do those things; you've got to learn them by doing them.

All memory techniques are aimed at enhancing declarative memory: What can I do, what do I know, and how can I declare it? Inattention is the most common cause of forgetting. As we mentioned if there's no encoding there's no retrieving. The number one rule for memory is: Pay attention, as we discussed in last lecture. Of course attention increases with interest, and varies with interest. Increase your areas of interest and you become more attentive, your memory is better. Even people with ADHD can learn and remember if they're interested in the topic. Take your time. As Milan Kundera says in his novel, "There is a secret bond between slowness and memory, between speed and forgetting."

Let's talk now about some general rules for enhancing your memory. In Lecture 12 we will cover memory techniques and systems to super power your memory and super charge it. Over the next few minutes we will cover how to sharpen sense memory, augment general memory in short-term memory, long-term memory, and working memory. Remember: The most important principle for improving your memory is focusing your attention on what you're trying to learn. That's why I spoke of attention in a previous lecture before we moved on to memory. Distraction in our time is the basis for information overload and for inattention.

You should start with sense memory because that's the brain's initial recording of physical sensations as they impinge on our sense organs. It can be iconic memory, what we see; echoic memory, what we hear; and in addition, what we touch, taste, and smell. Too often sensation occurs outside of awareness. I'm going to suggest exercises that can help you to enhance memory via heightening conscious awareness.

An example of this in the epigraph of the book *The Motorcycle Diaries of Che Guevara* where it's stated, "If you can see, look. If you can look, observe." Of course if you do that you're paying full attention and you're likely to remember. Jose Saramago, the famous Nobel Prize winning author, had an uncle who described what a bull is like when faced with a bullfighter this way: "He sees you, and then when he has seen you, he looks at you, and this time there is something different about it: he observes you." This is an example of paying full attention and remembering, just like the bull is going to remember certain things. A lot of times we go through life without remembering what we're doing. Have you ever noticed someone looking at a watch and then a second later you ask them, "What time is it?" and they look again? Why would that be? Didn't they just look? Don't they remember exactly what they saw? It's an example of where we are not paying attention to our sensory input.

Here are some exercises to sharpen the special senses of taste and smell. You recall in the earlier lecture, we went over some sensory exercises for vision, hearing, hand dexterity, and peripersonal space. Here we will take up exercises for the special senses of taste and smell. Let's start off by taking a number of spices at random and setting them out on a table. Close your eyes and identify by smell alone such things as oregano, mint, minced onion, sage, sweet basil, orange, cumin, and black pepper, a whole array. Olfaction sensory fibers connect by the way directly to the brain they no intermediary, it doesn't go through the thalamus. This is why it's the most direct point of sensory input. Now combine this knowledge with identifying spices in a meal that you are eating. Ask the cook, What did they put in? If you're in a restaurant try to find out. When you're making a meal with spices, try not putting the spices in a certain half. Do you taste the difference? Of course you do. Cooking is one of the best ways of enhancing you're your sensory memory along with other things like general episodic memory and frontal lobe—this is really the real example of frontal lobe coordinating things so that everything just right. Just like the CEO of the kitchen if you will, so that everything is ready on time. The older you are the more difficult it is to learn to cook, but start wherever. I started cooking only 10 years ago. I'm certainly not a chef but I think I can make a decent meal.

Memory is short-term and long-term memory. Short-term memory is maintained through active rehearsal, you keep going over something. It eventually gets into long-term memory and you have the storage of information. Every day of our lives we strengthen this through active efforts to learn new information through reading or taking courses like this one.

A powerful short-term memory strengthening exercises would be a simple exercise that's a predictor of math, and reading proficiency, attention, concentration, sequencing, and auditory and visual short-term memory. It's called the digit span exercise. We'll do it first with auditory recall. Read into the recorder a series of 5, 6, 7 and 8 digit strings. You'll probably want to group them so that all the 5-digit strings are together, the 6-digit strings are together, and so on. Now put them aside for while and clear you mind. Several hours later listen to the lists, pause, and then write down as many of those strings that you can recall. Then play the recording to check for accuracy.

You can do this visually by writing those lists on a piece of paper. Write the list, turn them face down, look at them quickly one at a time, and then try to remember the sequence as you saw. You can check at the end by turning them face up again.

There are benefits for doing both visual and auditory span. First of all it's a quick test of whether you are a visual or auditory learner. It focuses attention and it focuses concentration. A digit span can be increased by practice—you start at 5 and work your way up. A normal adult digit span is between 5 and 7. It's very interesting that one number per year of age is normal, starting at about 3, so a 2 year old can remember 2, a 3 year old can remember 3, etc. The average digit span of adults in other words is that of a 7-year-old child! You have to work on it to build it up.

The important principle is a principle called chunking, from the paper "The Magical Number Seven, Plus or Minus Two" by George Miller, who was a Princeton psychologist. He found that if you chunk the numbers so that you take long strings and break them up into parts. That's what we do with telephone number. We remember the first 3 numbers, then we have a space, then we remember the last 4 numbers. The brain doesn't spontaneously encode into short-term memory more than 7 items. If you want to improve your digit span you have to practice it.

Why bother to practice and lengthen the digit span, you might ask? It seems trivial, doesn't it? It's not something most of us do but what's happening is that the digit span is a predictor of math and reading and enhanced performance in attention, concentration, sequencing and auditory and visual short-term memory. Don't be fooled by the apparent simplicity of this exercise. This is a powerful way of improving brain function in multiple areas.

Short-term memory needs to be in active rehearsal in order to be moved to long-term memory. Attention must be focused on material. If attention is disrupted by distraction, like when somebody asks you a question, then we lose the track of it. But rehearsal alone isn't sufficient. Depth of processing is required. Rote repetition is not as effective as working with the information. Memorization of dates, for instance, is not as effective as writing an essay on what happened on that particular date. Depth of processing increases the web of connections among stored memories, so in other words it increases neuronal connections that we've talked about throughout these lectures.

There's also an importance of repeated testing. Tests should include old as well as new material. For instance, do you remember those ornery professors from college who unexpectedly subjected you to pop quiz? Most annoying of all were those who went back and retested you on things you had already been tested on. You say, Professor we've already gone through all that before. Well it turns out those professors were right, they were on to something. Repeated testing is more effective for long-term learning than additional study. That's from research done by from Jeffrey Karpicke and Henry Roediger at Purdue University, described first in *Science*. Practicing retrieval during tests results in greater learning than study alone. It's better to go back and retest than it is to just keep studying the same things over and over. Even after the item has been learned the best way of remembering it is by retesting. Why? Well the neuronal networks, called cell assemblies by Canadian psychologist Donald Hebb, are strengthened each time the memory is retrieved. It's similar to physical training, if you think about it. After you build up a muscle or muscle group you have to keep exercising it or it will undergo the disuse atrophy that we talked about earlier. Similar results have been found in my own field of neurology. I teach medical students, they remembered more about neurological illnesses when they were repeatedly tested rather than the usual sequence of learning it, cramming it in overnight, and so forth. That's the way it should be; as a neurologist they don't know when they're going to see a certain thing so they don't learn a certain disease and sort of forget about it because they have to go one to other things. This has to be part of their permanent repertoire and the only way to do that is to be retested on it. As patients come in over the years, that's the form of retesting that they'll be exposed to.

Short-term memory is often sufficient to just rehearse a phone number, dial it, and forget it. Any storage of information you may want to mull over, manipulate it, you have to do so. Put it in your mind, you mentally rehearse the term, such as for instance the items on a grocery list you compare them to what you remember in your cabinets at home. That's memory, but it's a special kind of memory. It's called working memory. It's when you manipulate information in your memory. You're using a special form of memory, you're not just going back and linking things up one after another instead you're moving them around. If I ask you a certain thing like name all the players on your baseball team. You name them and that's general memory. But if I ask you to give them to me by which position they're in or who came on the team first, this sort of thing, then that's working memory.

From our discussion in this lecture of general memory we're going to move on in our next lecture to this most important memory process of all, the working memory. Which I'm going to mention to you is so important, that we can say that it is probably the most important element to keep sharp throughout our lifespan in order to optimize brain function. Thank you.

# Exercising Your Working Memory
## Lecture 7

**Our intelligence is related to our ability to transfer information from working memory to long-term memory. ... In fact, the greater the working memory, the higher the verbal score on the Scholastic Aptitude Test and ... IQ tests.**

Working memory is central to the most important mental operation carried out by the human brain: manipulating stored information. Working memory involves a relatively small number of items that are simultaneously kept track of, and the number of items and the ease of recall varies from one person to another. The good news is that working memory can be improved by practice.

First let's look at an example of when we might use working memory in our everyday lives. Perhaps you want to throw a dinner party composed of people who may or may not be compatible. Imagine a group of 12 people composed of neighbors, coworkers from your job, coworkers from your husband's job—a mixed group. You have to mentally review people, their personalities, and your impression of them to plan a dinner party that will be harmonious.

What are the brain areas involved with working memory? This type of memory is really the key function of the frontal areas. Think of a scratch pad maintained in the frontal lobes that the rest of the brain can then consult and become familiar with over time. Since working memory depends primarily on the prefrontal cortex, it varies with age. Young children have difficulty organizing themselves, keeping their attention focused, and managing multiple things at a time.

If working memory is a scratch pad, then long-term memory is its filing system. A transfer occurs from working memory into long-term memory, where knowledge is organized into complex concepts. Our intelligence is related to our ability to transfer information from working memory to long-term memory. Information in our working memory is known as cognitive load. If that load is exceeded, information isn't encoded and cannot be transferred to long-term memory. Technology, especially the Internet, increases cognitive load and interferes with the formation of long-term memory.

So let's start building our working memory with an easy example: backward digit span. This is similar to the earlier exercise we did, but this time if you hear or read 1234, instead of 1234, you respond with 4321. Try it for 4-digit numbers, 5-digit numbers, 6-digit numbers, and maybe even 7-digit numbers. After doing numbers, try spelling words backward. "World" is D-L-R-O-W. Progress to "hospital," "democracy" (which is a tough one)—and if you really get good, try a word like "irresponsibility." Always work on maintaining or building up your skill level.

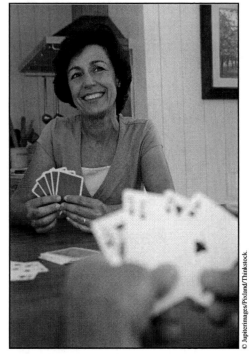

**Card games are great exercise for your working memory.**

© Jupiterimages/Pixland/Thinkstock.

Here is another exercise for you to try. Put out some coins—dimes, nickels, and quarters. If someone were to ask you how you would total these, you would more than likely first count all of, say, the nickels; then the dimes; and then the quarters. If you really want to test your working memory, count them in such a way that you have to keep a separate running total of each type of coin. Another way to do it is to total the coins in terms of their value. Keep them on separate tracks—so if you have 2 quarters, you have 50 cents; 3 nickels are 15 cents; and 2 dimes are 20 cents—and then at the end, add them up. You should start with 2 types of coins and then work your way up, if you can, to 4. This is very difficult.

Recreational games are also good exercise for your working memory. The card game bridge forces you to remember and manipulate cards in play while you're also exercising your general memory by remembering how that particular hand did the last time you were playing. On tests of working memory and reasoning, bridge players outperform people who don't play bridge. Poker, incidentally, is just as good. Card counting is probably the most quintessential example of multitasking in some ways, but it's mostly a test of working memory.

**If working memory is a scratch pad, then long-term memory is its filing system.**

Notice that the exercises in working memory also involve creativity. They involve looking at things in great detail and being able to put them together. They also require heightened alertness and awareness, as well as the discovery of linkages between the past and the present. Working memory exercises can be a great learning and refreshing tool. ∎

## Suggested Reading

Gluck, Mercado, and Meyers, *Learning and Memory.*

Schacter, *The Seven Sins of Memory.*

# Exercising Your Working Memory

## Lecture 7—Transcript

Welcome back. In this lecture, we'll talk about working memory and what you can do to improve it. Working memory is central to the most important mental operation carried out by the human brain: manipulating stored information. Let me give you a few examples. Imagine Robert, a college sophomore, getting ready for his 9:30 psychology class. Several errands along the way he plans to do. He wants to drop off laundry, pick up several Lady Gaga concert tickets and visit the ATM machine. He mentally pictures the locations of these stops and plots out the most efficient to get there. He finally gets to the psychology class but finds a note on the door announcing a relocation for the day. Robert quickly reorganizes his itinerary. It's now on the third floor front in another building instead of basement. He arrives just in time. He recalls subject of last lecture, opens computer, and checks notes from last class, and gets started. Just as he was listening he remembers it's his sister's birthday and goes online to send off a computer birthday card. Around this time the professor singles Robert out and asks him a question. He puts everything else temporarily out of mind as he answers the question. After class, Robert mentally calculates what each person owes for the concert tickets and he also works out in his mind an itinerary of each ticket buyer's location and how to get there most efficiently.

To keep track of this Robert had to do a lot of things, juggle lots of information, had to integrate it. At various times he was setting goals, task switching, inhibiting habitual responses, and working with unexpected developments, such as remembering his sister's birthday and sending that birthday card. Robert is keeping a lot of things in mind at once, you can think of him as a juggler keeping many balls in the air while actually holding only one or two at any one moment.

Let me give you another example: This is a lost key. Remember the last time you lost a key? Imagine that you can't find your key in the morning when you're getting ready to go to work. The key to your automobile. You look for it in a very systematic way. You try to remember when did last see it? If the key wasn't at that place, you looked elsewhere while avoiding places you already looked. You remained focused on the goal of finding the key.

You juggle all kinds of information. You ignored distractions—if someone calls you say, I don't really have time to talk right now I'm lost something important. You concentrated instead on related information: Where do I customarily put the key? Why isn't it there now? Do I have an extra key, and if I do where is it? You then remembered suddenly the consequences the last time you were late for work. You end the key search and call a co-worker and ask her to pick you up on her way to the office.

As these examples show working memory involves a relatively small number of items that are simultaneously kept track of and the number of items and the ease of recall varies from one person to another. The most important message I have today is that working memory can be improved by practice. You might ask, Why bother to improve working memory? For several reasons. One of which is working memory is linked with IQ and it's the first to decline with aging. There's also different encoding in the brain than general memory. This is a working lecture in which we will learning about working memory through exercises and how you can improve your working memory.

Let's start with an easy example. Let's start with what's called backward digit span. Remember in a previous lecture we got numbers 1234 and we tried to remember them in that sequence? This time we're going to do them backwards so instead 1234 would be 4321.Do that for 4-digit numbers, 5-digit numbers, 6-digit numbers, and maybe even 7-digit numbers. Try to give them backwards, try to build up your ability to do that. After doing numbers try doing words spelled backwards. World is D-L-R-O-W, move on to hospital, democracy—which is a tough one, you have to keep those letters in your mind—once you get good at that move on to a word like irresponsibility. Establish the word length that you're comfortable with and can manage.

Next we're going from single words to sequenced information. Take any sequence of information, maybe a sports team, the hit recordings by a singer, and shift the information around according to dates, alphabetical listing, whatever. Let's try it with the U.S. presidents starting with Obama and going back to Franklin Delano Roosevelt. So we have Barack Obama, George Walker Bush, Bill Clinton, George Herbert Walker Bush, Ronald

Reagan, Jimmy Carter, Gerald Ford, Richard Nixon, Lyndon Johnson, John Fitzgerald Kennedy, Dwight Eisenhower, Harry Truman, and Franklin Delano Roosevelt. When you do that, reciting that list as I've just done, it is a test of general memory, which is the topic of our next lecture. Let's convert that list into a test of working memory: Name only the Democratic presidents starting with Obama and going back forward. Do that now, time yourself without writing anything down—name them. Barack Obama, Bill Clinton, Jimmy Carter, Lyndon Johnson, John Fitzgerald Kennedy, Harry Truman, and Franklin Delano Roosevelt. Now let's do the Republican presidents. We'll skip Obama of course and move back to George W. Bush. Name all of the Republican presidents—time yourself. We have of course George W. Bush, George H. W. Bush, Ronald Reagan, Gerald Ford, Richard Nixon, and Dwight Eisenhower.

In order to do those 2 exercises you had to perform the following steps and functions. Recall all of the presidents in order but suppress certain names depending on political party. There was no need to rearrange anything. Here is a more challenging working memory exercise: Name the presidents in alphabetical order between Obama and Franklin Delano Roosevelt. It takes quite a bit longer to think about it. George Bush, George Bush, Jimmy Carter, Bill Clinton, Dwight Eisenhower, Gerald Ford, Lyndon Johnson, John Fitzgerald Kennedy, Richard Nixon, Barack Obama, Ronald Reagan, Franklin Delano Roosevelt, and Harry Truman. Notice how much more difficult the last exercise was compared to the first two? In this one you had to do more than just suppress the democrat or republican, you had to mentally re-arrange things.

There are some everyday examples of working memory, for instance getting together a dinner party composed of people who may or may not be compatible. Imagine 12 people composed of neighbors, coworkers from your job, coworkers from your husband's job, a mixed group—you have to figure things out in such a way that you can mentally reviewing people, their personalities, your impression of them you can plan a dinner party that would be harmonious. Two other examples: How about running through your mind a new recipe before you begin making it? This is an excellent test for working memory and I recommend it highly. Another is recalling and pondering all of your past discussions about office routine with an employee.

Word processing, if you think about it, provides a metaphor for working memory. When working on 2 documents you can shift back and forth from one and the other, keeping one open and on screen while keeping the other sort of in mind in another window. You can toggle from one to the other. If you were to forget one you would be suffering the equivalent of a loss in working memory. If you are interrupted during a talk with an employee and forget your point, that's called the interference effect, which is essentially a failure in working memory.

A bridge game is an excellent way of testing and exercising your working memory. Remembering and manipulating cards in play or you can also be exercising your general memory by remembering how that particular hand did the last time you were playing.

Let's talk a little bit about the brain areas having to do with working memory. This is really the key area, and key function, of the frontal areas. Let me tell you how we discovered that. In the 1930s Carlyle Jacobsen, a physiologist, studied the effects of injuries to the frontal lobes on monkeys. The injuries were such that if you put food in 1 of 2 trays, the monkey would look at it and obviously reach for that food. But later if you put a curtain down, kept it down for a few seconds then raised the curtain, the monkey would not remember which tray had the food. A short delay was creating a failure in remembering where the food was. These were the monkeys with frontal lobe injuries, they couldn't point to the dish where they had previously seen the food.

Subsequent research by another doctor, Joaquin Fuster and others, established that parts of the prefrontal cortex, the area up front that we've talked so much about already in previous lectures, are devoted to retaining information despite delay. The monkey was unable to remember which tray the food was in because there was this delay. Think of a scratch pad maintained in the frontal lobes that the rest of the brain can then consult and become familiar with over time. Now you might suspect because of what we've said in cerebral geography, the left frontal cortex is important for verbal working memory; the parietal lobe is too but mostly the frontal. This is consistent with our knowledge that left hemisphere mediates language. The right frontal cortex is concerned with visual-spatial processing as we've discussed before on the lecture on cerebral geography.

Since working memory depends primarily on the prefrontal cortex it varies with age. Working memory, for instance, is very poor in children. As a result, young children have a difficult time organizing themselves, keeping their attention focused, managing more than one thing at a time. This is what they have parents for, some people would say. The dorsolateral prefrontal cortex is especially important. It forms an internal representation or mental snapshots if you will, and helps you to retain focus such as when you look for that key.

If working memory is a scratch pad, long-term memory is its filing system. Long-term memory is unconscious. Working memory, however, is conscious. You're conscious of it all the time—just like Robert in the beginning of the lecture is conscious of all these things he's doing and planning, and using his working memory.

A transfer occurs from working memory into long-term memory. Long-term memory organizes knowledge into complex concepts or schemas. It's aided in this by working memory. The key point is that our intelligence is related to our ability transfer information from working memory to long-term memory. Students with low working memory skills are prone to misunderstandings and mistakes in class and on tests. In fact, the greater the working memory, the higher the verbal score on the Scholastic Aptitude Test (SATs) and they score higher on IQ tests. They also do better on standard nonverbal tests. Why would you think they would do better on nonverbal tests? If you remember back to the types of tests I'm talking about, these can be very difficult tests based on the number of factors that must be kept in mind. When we say kept in mind, we mean in working memory.

Since working memory is so important I'm going to spend the rest of the lecture giving you some exercises you can take to improve it. But first some things to keep in mind: Distraction is the greatest enemy of working memory. Distraction interferes with consolidation, which is what memory is all about. Consolidation is the first step in memory formation. In fact when you take classic memory tests are actually working memory tests. I sometimes ask people I'm evaluation to remember 4 items and then I ask them about them after a 4-minute delay. I might say something like, apple,

Mr. Johnson, charity, and tunnel. They will repeat it and then I'll ask them about it 4-minuntes later they have to keep it in their working memory.

Information in our working memory is known as cognitive load. If load is exceeded information isn't encoded and cannot be transferred to long-term memory and concepts of course aren't formed. Technology especially the Internet increases cognitive load and interferes with the formation of long-term memory. In the last lecture we talked about the penalties exacted by multitasking. Our working memory is exceeded, we're perpetually distracted, and we show many of the subtle signs of ADHD.

Today we're going to concentrate on how to improve you're working memory. There are various ways to improve working memory. First control multitasking, which causes a frontal lobe bottleneck, overworks the frontal lobes, interferes with metacognition, which is remaining aware of your cognitive performance. First we're going to talk about the Semantic Fluency Test. In 1 minute name as many animals as you can. No repetition is allowed so you have to use working memory to mentally eliminate any you have already named. Try that; see how many you get in 1 minute. Time yourself. Now 17–20 is a desirable score.

A second test is called the Lexical Fluency Test. In 1 minute name as many words as you can beginning with the letter S. Try that. Then repeat it with the letter F. You can't use proper names, just regular words. Aim for something between 20–25, which would be a good initial score.

Another way of testing working memory is with coins which I'm going to show you now. I'm going to put out some coins—dimes, nickels, and quarters. If someone were to ask you how you would total these, you would more than likely pick up one at a time of say the nickels, get them all and say there's 4 or 5 nickels here. Then you would do the dimes and say there's 6 or 7 dimes here, then the same with quarters and pennies. If you really want to test your working memory you would do each of them separately in such a way that you would have to keep a separate running total of what each one is. How many there are in total. Another way to do it is to total them in terms of what they actually come to. So if you have 2 quarters you have 50 cents, if you have 3 quarters you have 75 cents, if you have 2 dimes you have 20 cents. Keep them on separate tracks, separate files if you will, and then at the end put them together. And of course you can check your accuracy by as you pick up the coins you can put them to one side and then later you can check how well you did.

Now to try that yourself you have to do that with 2 at the same time, probably dimes and nickels, and then work your way up if you can to 4 denominations. Most people can only handle 2 at the beginning. The coin counting test is hard. Start with 2 and work up to 4, and as I said make it even harder by totaling the amount. There is no way to do any of these exercises without focused attention. That's why we spoke of attention in an earlier lecture. The goal in each of the fluency tests is to activate the frontal executive circuits.

Here is another working memory exercise you can do right now called the N-Back test. You do it with a pack of cards. Take the deck of cards after they've been shuffled and you pick a trigger card—let's say it's a queen. Then you start turning the cards over until you come to the card you were looking for, the queen. Then you remember what was there 2 cards before the queen. In this case it's the joker. After you get good at that you can go back 3 cards. That causes a very good exercise in working memory.

Here's another working memory test: Read numbers into a voice recorder and then put it away. Come back and listen to recording listening for a randomly selected number. When you hear the number, stop the recording and write down the number you heard 2 previously. Then reverse your recording and check your accuracy.

Suppose you have neither a deck of cards or a voice recorder handy at the moment, here is a way to do it with a book. Most books as you've probably noted have pagination in the upper right hand corner. I found one, it happens to be one of my own books, with pagination at the bottom that enables you write numbers on the right hand page, one number per page. Generate them at random; make a whole list of them. Then when you have 30 or 40 of them, you can fan through them looking for a specific number—let's say 3. When you come to 3, then you remember what you saw 2 pages earlier or 3 pages earlier. This is another example where you can use.

Here is another test: Write down the following names: Fred, Stacy, Richard, Stanly, Ida, and Ed. Recite the list, now that of course is general memory. Then recite it backwards. Then recite in alphabetical order. And finally recite it according to word length because the names have different numbers of letters. Ed is 2, Ida is 3, Fred is 4, Stacy is 5, Stanly is 6, and Richard is 7.

Working memory for designs can also be done. In 4 minutes draw as many original abstract designs as you can. This is something that can't be named, it's just abstract. The key is to not have any repetitions. Recreational games are also good in terms of working memory. Dominoes and bridge boost working memory. On tests of working memory and reasoning bridge players out perform people who don't play bridge. Poker, incidentally, is just as good. There are differences between poker and bridge of course. One of which is the personality; loners and people who don't tend to be interacting too much with people tend to enjoy poker more. Others who are more social tend to enjoy bridge. That's not a cut at anybody who plays poker it's just something to keep in mind when you select the working memory recreational game you're going to take. Incidentally when talking about cards, card counting is probably the most quintessential example of multitasking in some ways but mostly a test of working memory.

Now here's a quick test of your working memory. Ready? What was the last movie you saw? That question might be easy to answer if you rarely go to the movies. You sort of go into long-term memory and say, Well, I guess a year ago I saw a movie. But if you go frequently, you may running a little mental movie of your own, thinking of movie companions, your usual habits (movies on weekends only, during the week, with lunch or dinner, all these various things. And suddenly you're running through your working memory all kinds of information not directly related to movies.

What other things can you do to enhance working memory? Take up activities and games as I mentioned, that involve working memory. I mentioned bridge and poker; chess is a great one. Also at odd moments mentally manipulate such things as the names of the players on your favorite team.

Notice that the exercises in working memory also involve creativity. They involve the powers of observation, looking at things in great detail and being able to put them together. Also heightened alertness and awareness, if you're not alert and aware you're not able to do any of these exercises. It's also the discovery of linkages between the past and the present. You also remember in the past we talked about the future memory, which is linking the past to the present to the future and is enhanced when you're doing a working memory exercise.

Working memory exercises can be a great learning and refreshing tool. Review and then recite the states for instance. Go from east to west, then west to east, or according to their founding dates.

To summarize this lecture, we've discussed one of the most distinguishing characteristics of the human brain, mainly maintaining information, keeping it in mind, while turning our attention to something else. As we discussed before increasing our working memory leads to an IQ increase as well. Finally, by improving working memory we exercise our frontal lobes, our most highly evolved brain structure.

# Putting Your Senses to Work
## Lecture 8

It's been shown that the retrieval context should equal the encoding context. There's an amusing experiment done with a diving club. Some of the people in the diving club memorized a list of numbers while they were underwater, and the others learned the number list while they were on land. It was found later that the ones that were tested in the same situation, either underwater or on land, did better than those who learned underwater and were quizzed on land or vice versa.

Throughout history, many imaginative techniques have been suggested to improve memory. In this lecture, we will discuss some contemporary examples of powerful ways of supercharging your memory. First, let's review a few general principles. The first principle is focus: Pay attention to what you're trying to memorize. Second, search for meaning in the information; of course, this meaning will vary according to circumstance and to you as an individual. Use as many sensory faculties as possible—see it, hear it, and touch it. You can also put information in the form of an image. The clearer the image, the more likely you are to remember it. Third, you can also create a system of memory pegs, which we'll discuss below.

Since paying attention is the most fundamental rule for improving memory, here are some quick warm-up exercises to sharpen attention—apply them just before memorizing. Rapidly scan a few pictures and then describe what you saw. Then look back and check for accuracy. Also try drawing something and then verbally describing what you have drawn.

Now that you're warmed up, let's learn how to use memory pegs. My personal method is to memorize a dozen neighborhood sites. For me, they are (1) my home, (2) a library, (3) a photo store, and so on. I rehearse them for a long time, forward and backward; they are very clear in my mind. Then I take each of the items I want to remember, like on a grocery list, and compose a vivid bizarre image of that item on a site that I have in my memory. For instance, if I'm going to the store to get some soda, I might see a soda can reading a book in front of my home.

Make up your own list of places in your neighborhood. You could use your house or apartment, but I advise using the neighborhood because it's more expansive. Practice the list until you can rapidly name it and see it. Then place your memory items in these pegs.

Now let's move on to memorizing nonverbal material, which is a lot tougher. The key concept here is to increase your memory for nonverbal material without resorting to words or any type of internal dialogue. This calls on the right hemisphere, which handles activities like processing visual-spatial information. Jigsaw puzzles, for instance, are great stimulators of the right hemisphere.

Let's practice a few right hemisphere exercises. Close your eyes and envision the room that you are in. Open your eyes and check for accuracy. Repeat this

## Exercise Your Brain with Television!

Here are exercises involving visual sequences that you can practice at home.

- Watch a television drama while recording it, and then replay it in your mind scene by scene. Watch it again to check the correctness of your memory.

- Do the same with a documentary: Mentally replay the program with its interviews and commentary. Then watch it again, and check how well you did.

- Watch a basketball or hockey game while recording it. After a score occurs, review in your mind what you think you observed—then play the program back and see how clearly you remembered the scoring situation.

exercise, paying attention to small details—like the number of magazines on a table. During the day, carry a camera with you and take pictures of various scenes. You can check later what you can remember and the accuracy of your recall.

**We are visual creatures: The more vivid, dramatic, and bizarre the image, the more likely we are to remember it.**

Here are some pattern exercises that enhance right hemisphere functioning. Draw free-form designs, memorize them, and reproduce them—this is not only a test of memory but also of eye-hand coordination and motor memory. Memorize and sketch the layout of a room or the seating arrangements at a dinner table. Here's a personal example of a waiter in one of my favorite restaurants. He never writes anything down, so I asked him how he does this. He told me he first visually memorizes the menu. As the customer orders, he substitutes that item on the menu with a mental picture of the customer. In the kitchen he reconverts from the picture to the menu item.

What do all these various memory exercises have in common? They force you to pay attention to what you're trying to learn. They also encourage you to emphasize a visual format. We are visual creatures: The more vivid, dramatic, and bizarre the image, the more likely we are to remember it. Using memory techniques will hone your attentional abilities, help you link your memory with cognitive processes like learning and creativity, and may help stave off Alzheimer's disease. Developing a superpower memory also links you to larger cultural currents. If you remember more, you experience more—so enriching your memory can enrich your life! ■

## Suggested Reading

Restak, *Mozart's Brain and the Fighter Pilot.*

# Putting Your Senses to Work
## Lecture 8—Transcript

Welcome back. Throughout history many imaginative memory techniques have been suggested to improve memory. Today we will discuss and try a few of them.

The inventor of mnemonics, which is the art and science of memory, is reputed to be a Greek poet Simonides, who lived between c. 556–468 B.C. Cicero describes Simonides' method in his account of a banquet in the house of a man named Scopas. Simonides was hired to write and recite a poem praising Scopas, but only half of the poem praised Scopas. The other half was devoted to the divine twins Castor and Pollux. Scopas became angry and wanted to pay only half of the fee so they were having some negotiations about this. A message was delivered to the hall that 2 men outside wished to speak with Simonides. Those 2 men were Castor and Pollux, who had come to pay Simonides in a very special way for his speech praising them. Within seconds the roof of the banquet hall collapsed killing everyone inside. Simonides used his remarkable memory to identify each of the mangled bodies by what came to be called the method of place.

Simonides pictured in his mind where each guest had been seated. In this way he identified each of the bodies. Here is Cicero's explanation of what Simonides had done: He inferred that persons desiring to train this faculty must select places and form mental images of the things they wish to remember and store those images in places, so that the order of the places will preserve the order of the things, and the images of the things will denote the things themselves, and we shall employ the places and images respectively as a wax writing-tablet and the letters written on it.

Simonides art was based on 2 simple concepts: places and images. Quintilian, who lived between A.D. 35–96, redefined this concept by describing an architectural technique (and that's the term he used) for imprinting the memories within a large building. Here is how it works: You physically walk through the building's numerous rooms and remember all of the ornaments and furnishings that you encounter and see. You then convert each idea to be remembered into an image. You then mentally walk through the building and deposit each of these images in the order of the ornaments and furnishings you have previously memorized. This method still works today and is used by memory virtuosos who perform seemingly impossible feats of memory.

We are going to discuss some contemporary examples of these ancient and powerful ways of super charging your memory but first, a few principles. All memory techniques are based on a few principles, the first of which is focusing, paying attention to what you're trying to memorize. Secondly, searching for meaning in the information, and of course this meaning will vary according to circumstance and according to your own background. Use as many sensory faculties as possible—seeing it, hearing it, and touching it. You also put information in the form of an image and that's the most important part. The clearer the image the more likely you will be to remember it. You make that image distinct and clear, crystal clear. You also create a system of memory pegs based on your life experience.

Here are some additional suggestions given to me by Mark Gluck, who is a memory researcher at Rutgers University and has written a textbook on memory. He says create associations. He gives us an example of Ag, which is the symbol for silver in the periodic table. Ag comes from Latin *argentum*, which means silver. Argentina was named Argentina because it was thought to be filled with silver, but not that much has been found there. So this is a method of association. He also practice and drill, as we did as children with states, planets, and multiplication tables. Also reading the information aloud is helpful. The other senses too as I mentioned, holding it in hand or touching it. Try to reduce overload. You can use Post-It notes or other things for routine things that you want to be free of as you try to concentrate and focus on the things you're trying to memorize. You also get involved with this form of time-travel, you remember when and circumstances where you learned something. Also get adequate sleep, as we talked in the earlier lecture there are a lot of people in the country right now that have problems sleeping and don't get adequate sleep. Part of that is relaxing and not forcing memorization. Distract yourself and let your brain operate at its own pace. Use rhymes or songs as mentioned earlier.

Now for some specific memory techniques. First, look for ways of making the material meaningful. Here's a test: Recall these numbers in their exact order 1, 4, 9, 1, 6, 2, 5, 3, 6, 4, 9, 6, 4, 8, 1. Most people can manage about 7 of those 15 numbers. Let's see if I can do better. I'll close my eyes and see if I can do a little better. 1, 2—1, 4, 9, 1, 6, 2, 5, 3, 6, 4, 9, 6, 4, 8, 1. I think I did fairly well, I put one in early that wasn't there but I got the rest of it ok. How did I do that? First convert them into single digits and study them for a moment: 1, 4, 9, 1, 6, 2, 5, 3, 6, 4, 9, 6, 4, 8, 1. One observation will enable you to recite them rapidly and without error, as I think I did. Do you see what it is? They can be grouped to represent the squares of the numbers 1–9: 1, 4, 9, 16, 25, 36, 49, 64, 81. Granted, there was a little trickery there. Not every number sequence lends itself to such a quick fix. When it doesn't, you have to create your own grouping method. Look for ways of chunking, just like telephone numbers 202-362-0777 we don't say 2023620777. There's an historical example of chunking is Mozart's memorization of Miserere, written by Gregorio Allegri. The Vatican was the owner of the manuscript for this and they forbad publication. Mozart heard it only twice and then was able to write it out, which is considered to be a marvelous example of music. But musicians say the work is quite conventional and it's not difficult to chunk large portions of the work around its standard features. In other words it's not necessary to memorize note by note. So Mozart combined special knowledge, efficient processing, and chunking.

You should look for personal associations as aids to improve your memory performance. K. Anders Ericsson, now at Florida State University, conducted an experiment which will show you the benefits of this. This was an experiment on the effect of practice on memory for numbers. He had a student who he calls S. F., who started with 7 numbers by practicing 1 hour 2–3 times per week. He then could go from 7 to 10 digits. Several hundred hours of practice led to more than 80 digits at 1 digit a second. How did he do this? Here is are the first few numbers of one of S. .F.'s 80-digit numbers that he memorized 3583493527222750045 … etc. Now if you try even the first 20 you're going to have trouble with it. It's hard to do. But S. F. had a method. Any guesses about what that method was based on? Let me give you a clue. S. F. was an avid cross-country runner. What he was doing was increasing his memory for number by associating them with running times for various track and field events. The first few numbers 358 is a very fast mile: 3 minutes and 58 seconds. For a 4-digit number he added split seconds: 3493, 3 minutes 49.3 secs. When trying to memorize something try to relate it to something you know or do, just like S. F. did. If you're a doctor maybe you'll think blood pressure, or pulse readings, or height and weight charts. Literally see in your mind's eye the material as clearly as possible.

When reviewing something you previously memorized try to duplicate the circumstances at the time you first learned it. It's been shown that the retrieval context should equal the encoding context. There's an amusing experiment done with a diving club. Some of the people in the diving club memorized a list of numbers while they were underwater, and the others learned the number list while they were on land. It was found later that the ones that were tested in the same situation, either underwater or on land, did better than those who learned underwater and were quizzed on land or vice versa. Also it's interesting that you can improve your memory by listening to the same type of background music. The point is that we remember best what we encode most clearly and vividly. Let's give you an example: suppose you're the type of person who leaves your umbrella at the office oftentimes. The next morning when you get up and it's raining you think, Oh my gosh, my umbrella's at the office. One of the ways to remember it is to associate one of the first things you do when you leave the office to going home with your umbrella. For example if you ride in an elevator, picture your umbrella pushing the button. That of course will cause you to look for your umbrella before you leave the office.

Words are memory boosters. Words prime the brain's visual areas. The resulting mental images make us more sensitive to what we're trying to memorize. This is called top-down processing—we've shown the picture in one of the earlier lectures where the upper part of the brain is controlling the limitations on the lower part, the sensory input. There's focusing from the top to the bottom, very focused and concentrated. As a Cheerios or Sprite experiment it was shown that by repeating the product's name to themselves, people were able quickly find those items hidden in pictures of a crowded supermarket shelf. Knowing the name for something helps you to find it quickly. For instance when you know the certain name for a plant and go out into a garden, you very quickly find it. The underlying theme is: Learn more, see more. Knowing the name for a concept helps you work with it. Learn more, do more.

In an experiment if people heard a letter said out loud it helped them find it among a string of other letters. Since learning new words is a key component to memory enhancement, try to learn as many new words as possible. If you do just 1 a day that's 365 words a year; 2 words it's double that and so forth. Learn a new word every day and keep the word in a journal. Today's word for me is sedulous: involving great care, effort, and persistence. And here's a sentence: She was sedulous and would work on a poem for years. It was written about an American poet.

How best to learn a new word? When attempting to memorize words learn the meaning of the word, the language of origin, and the root. Break the word into its component parts. Use the word in a sentence, as I just did. Pronounce the word and review its meaning. Spell the word to yourself and match it with its sound. Mentally picturing the word brings more brain structures into play. You want to bring as many senses into play as you can, listen to yourself saying it. This increases the linkages of word and its networks. And of course we talked in great detail about the networks of the brain can actually mirror the networks that you're trying to find in terms of knowledge.

I asked the winner of adult spelling bee for his secrets. He told me he made tapes of word for listening while commuting or jogging. He spent many hours of solitary word study. I used a similar multisensory method to preparing for an examination years ago. I was reading textbooks, writing, and also would dictate into a tape recorder that was used in those days. Then play them when I was driving around or otherwise unoccupied. I was then able to have two channels of input both having read it and having heard it. Sometimes I would sit home and read it while also listening to it at the same time so the two channels were working simultaneously.

Since paying attention is the most fundamental rule for improving memory here are some quick warm up exercises to sharpen attention—apply them just before memorizing. The visual one would be rapidly scanning pictures and describing what you saw. Then look back and check for accuracy. Or draw something and then verbally describe what you have drawn.

Now that you're warmed up, let's move on to memory techniques. The first book, the oldest memory book was written sometime between 80 and

82 B.C. It's called *Rhetorica ad Herennium*. It suggests skillfully linking items to be remembered with places and images, sort of like Simonides did at the banquet. Mentally place objects from a grocery list for instance, in locations in your living room. Imagine yourself walking through the room and observing the objects where you placed them.

My personal method is to memorize a dozen neighborhood sites. I rehearse them for a long time, forward and backward. Now I know them very clearly. Then I take each of the items I want to remember, like a grocery list, and compose a vivid bizarre image of that item on a site that I have in my memory. For instance, one of them is a library. So if I'm going to the store to get some Coca-Cola I might see a Coke can reading a book in front of my local library. My personal list is my home, #2 as I mentioned is a library, #3 is a photo store, supermarket, Georgetown Medical School, the main gates of Georgetown University, Café Milano, Key Bridge, the Iwo Jima Memorial, and Reagan Airport. I take the items I want to remember and I form an image as clear as I can make it. Then I place the images in front of those sites. I then mentally stroll along and see all these things, stroll along my memory pathway.

You have to make up your own personal list of places in your neighborhood. It could be in your house or apartment as well. I advise the neighborhood because it's more expansive; you're able to contain larger items in your imagination. You practice the list until you can rapidly name it and see it. Then you place memory items in these pegs.

We also have the story memory method. Try to remember these words for instance via a story: log, candy, shoe, tie pin, watch, ring, comb, and wallet. Try to come up with a story that is bizarre, wild, and vivid. Here is one: Image a log dressed as a man walking along the street eating a candy bar. He's quite dapper with Bruno Magli shoes and gold accessories (tie pin, a watch, a ring). Behind him is a pickpocket pretending to be combing his hair as he slip's his hand into the log's pocket and extracts the fat wallet.

The story method works for numbers but not as easily. Most of us use letters and words but not so much numbers. It's harder to mentally "see" numbers compared to envisioning objects. Here is the method I use to work with numbers from 0 to 10: 0 is hero, 1 is sun, 2 is shoe, 3 tree, 4 is door, 5 is hive, 6 is sticks, 7 is heaven, 8 is skate, 9 is vine, and 10 is hen. So whenever I see those numbers I substitute those images and visions of those. If I have a number like 2023627834, I repeat it using the above mnemonic to create a vivid story image. For instance to get the 202 imagine your favorite sports hero holding a shoe in each hand. How about a power saw reducing a tree to sticks for number 36? For 27 imagine an angel playing a shoe-shaped harp. For 834, imagine a skate shaped like a tree coursing over an ice pond and crashing into a barn door. That gives you all the numbers: 202 362 7834.

Take those words and those numbers and make up your own story. You will be associating and elaborating—the 2 most basic memory techniques as we said earlier on our lecture on association. Try associating something new with something you are already familiar with. I know a dermatologist whose name is Dr. Spot. It's not very difficult to remember his name because Dr. Spot suggests the skin, suggests dermatology. Others are not so easy.

Use elaboration, give meaning to what you are trying to memorize. Devise a sentence or a code. While in medical school for instance we had to learn the cranial nerve starting with the olfactory nerve and going all the way down to the 12th nerve the hypoglossal nerve. We had this mnemonic: On old Olympus's towering tops a Finn and German vied at hops. The planetary sequence can be remembered by the mnemonic: My very educated mother just sent us nine pizzas. That's for Mercury, Venus, Earth, Mars, Jupiter, Saturn, Uranus, Neptune, and Pluto.

A highly recommend source for memory techniques involving verbal material is *The Memory Book*, it's been out now for 40 or more years, by Harry Lorayne and Jerry Lucas. It's a classic; it's highly recommend in terms of using kind of the method I'm describing now.

Now let's move on to memorizing nonverbal material. This is a lot tougher. The key concept here is to increase your memory for nonverbal material without resorting to words or any type of internal dialogue. This will involve calling on the right hemisphere, and the key concept here is to shift your brain's processing from primarily left hemisphere activities like reading and writing to right hemisphere activities like processing visual-spatial information. Jigsaw puzzles are great stimulators of the right hemisphere.

In fact I want to read a quote to you from the novelist Margaret Drabble and what she has to say about jigsaw puzzles. "I think one of the reasons I am drawn to these puzzles is precisely because they have no verbal content; they exercise a different area of the brain, bring different neurons and dendrites into play. Like many people, I use the word-based, verbal left side of my brain too much." That's what we're aiming to do, what she just described.

Here are some right hemisphere exercises. Close your eyes and envision the room that you are in right now, watching this video. Open your eyes and check for accuracy. Repeat with attention paid to small details like the number of magazines on a table. During the day carry a camera and take pictures and check later what you can remember and the accuracy of your recall.

Other right hemisphere processes and exercises include tangrams. This is an ancient Chinese puzzle game involving 7 geometric pieces, which can be placed into hundreds of distinct figures. You can use them to make a bird or a woman pouring tea. Think of one of these figures and try to form it by manually arranging the 7 pieces. Next mentally arrange the pieces and memorize the arrangement. Be sure to memorize it, repeat it later and see if you can do it. The tangram involves gaining a sense of the feel of the geometric figures in the hand. That's one of the reasons many sets are made of fine woods. As you move the pieces around, your brain encodes the configuration and unconsciously manipulates it in mental space. As you play with this game you hone your 3-D memory.

Asian art, Tibetan art particularly, Tibetan Buddhist pictures and paintings were created with the art of visualization and memory in mind. Devotees studied the paintings until they could envision images in great detail. They believed visualization prepared their minds to assume the attributes of the beings portrayed in the paintings. Today we would emphasize the memory enhancing properties of these pictures for non- verbal concepts. Envision the scene as vividly as possible that you've seen on these pictures. Open your eyes and see what you missed. Close your eyes and see it again. If Asian art doesn't interest you study any of the works of Vermeer, Canaletto, or the Dutch masters known for finely detailed images. Study the works closely and with great intensity. Close your eyes and recall all the details you can.

Pay attention to one sector of the painting, close your eyes and envision it and you should be able to see it with even greater detail.

Here are some exercises that involve patterns that enhance right hemisphere functioning. Draw free-form designs, memorize them and reproduce them. It's not only a test of memory but also of eye-hand coordination and motor memory. Memorize and sketch the layout of room or the seating arrangements at a dinner table. Here's a personal example that I happen to know right here in Washington. A waiter in one of my favorite restaurants never writes anything down. I asked him how he did this. He told me he first memorizes the menu. As the customer orders, he substitutes that item on the menu with mental picture of the customer. In the kitchen he re-converts from the picture to the menu item. If he forgets anything, he looks again at his internal picture of the customers arranged according to their places on the memorized menu.

Next are exercises involving visual sequences. Record a television drama and then replay it in your mind scene by scene. Watch it again and check for the correctness of your memory. Or you can record a documentary and mentally replay the program with its interviews and commentary. Watch it again and check how well you did. Watch a basketball or an ice hockey game while simultaneously recording it. After a score occurs, review in your mind what you observed and then play back and see if how clearly you remembered the scoring situation. Other memory exercises involve mental chess and short games of chess. Classic chess problems are a very good way of doing it because these are essentially chess puzzles. I'll talk a bit about puzzles in a later lecture. You can also voice record the first dozen moves of a short game, you don't want a long game of chess, and record it slowly and distinctly. Then set up the board and play it while listening to the recording. Mentally move the pieces not moving with your hand. If you lose clarity open your eyes and physically move the pieces up to that point in the game. When finished, replay game from memory.

You can also use sound as a memory aid. Have you noticed that poetry is easier to memorize than prose? The brain loves the repetitive sounds and rhymes. That's why metric poetry is easier to learn than non-metric poetry. In preliterate times messages were conveyed in rhyme. In *Genghis Khan and the Making of the Modern World,* Jack Weatherford the author describes the practice in Khan's army where everyone, including Khan himself was illiterate. Let me quote from that "The Mongol warriors used a set of fixed melodies and poetic styles into which various words could be improvised according to the meaning of the message. For a soldier, hearing the message was like learning a new verse to a song that he already knew." To ensure accurate memorization, the officers often composed their orders in rhyme.

What do all these various memory exercises have in common? They force you to pay attention to what you're trying to learn, inattention is the greatest contributor to poor memories. They encourage you to emphasize a visual format: We are visual creatures. The more vivid, dramatic, and bizarre the image the more likely we are to remember it. The benefits of using memory techniques they will hone your attentional abilities, they will help you link your memory with other cognitive processes such as learning and creativity, and it may help stave off Alzheimer's disease. You also have to remember that memory is individual but it's also cultural. As a cultural Darwinian once said, "What has been done, thought, written, or spoken is not culture; culture is only that fraction that is remembered." Here are the cultural benefits of using a memory technique to develop a super power memory: It links you to the larger cultural currents. If you remember more, you experience more. If you enrich your memory, you enrich your life.

Obviously memory involves more than simply facts. We respond emotionally to our memories. Think of 9/11 and you don't just remember where you were but also how you felt. In the next lecture we're going to discuss how we can use our emotions as a memory aid. Thank you.

# Enlisting Your Emotional Memory
## Lecture 9

If you wanted to decide whether someone is lying to you, would you sooner meet them face-to-face, or would you sooner talk to them on the telephone? ... Most people would respond they would sooner encounter the person face-to-face. They are convinced they could tell in an instant if the person was lying by doing such things as staring them in the eye. Actually, the telephone is better since emotional leakage is greater in the auditory than the visual sphere. The reason for that is from our earliest years, we've learned to control our facial expressions.

In this lecture, we look at an aspect of memory that we do not usually consider—emotional memory. Despite its importance, most of us have lost touch with how we experienced the world in the past. Let me give you an example. I recently went to my high school reunion. I noticed that I recognized some people but not others; I recognized some of my good friends more quickly. We began to reminisce about football games, dances, and whatnot. We remembered all the incidents and events, but the memories of the emotions that accompanied them were not as clear.

Emotional memory becomes increasingly elusive the further we dig into the past. To experience the loss of emotional memory, page through some personal pictures. Start with photos taken a few weeks ago and work your way back to photos from a few years ago. Emotional memory is associated with the right hemisphere processing. Patients with right hemisphere injuries can't detect emotions in other people's faces or voices. They have a general loss of emotional interpretive and expressive ability.

Let's try several sense memory exercises based on the principle that the more vivid the sense memory, the greater the chances of establishing emotional memory. Indeed, by trying one of these exercises, you can learn much about emotional perception and memory. You may be able to evoke, explore, and even revisit your emotions—but approach these exercises in the spirit of play. Not taking yourself too seriously will give you a greater chance of making the exercises work.

The first exercise involves a partner. Sit together on the floor, maybe 2 or 3 feet apart, knees crossed, facing each other. Ask the other person to close her eyes and think of an emotion that is very sad. She is not to make any facial movements; she is only supposed to think these thoughts. Study her face as she's thinking about this. Then have her clear her face and think of something neutral. Then have her think of something happy. Observe her carefully. After that's over, you switch roles and work through the exercise again—sad, neutral, happy.

Afterward, compare notes about what you were thinking and what you saw in each other's faces. Was there anything that you noticed in her face? And when she had her eyes open, was there anything you saw in her eyes? It's important here not to inhibit facial expression but to remain vulnerable. It's a very unusual opportunity to be able to learn what someone is actually thinking—because she's going to tell you—and then compare that to what you picked up while you were looking at her. You can compare the things that she picked up in your facial expression and your eyes that you didn't in hers, and vice versa. The aim is for you to participate in her experience and for her to participate in yours.

The second exercise involves olfaction, which is the surest sense for enhancing emotional memory. Smell and taste are evocative because of the direct connection of olfactory nerve with the brain's limbic system. Invite some friends to your home, and have each of them bring something with a distinctive, pleasing smell: fresh cookies, sandalwood, mowed grass. Line the items up and have each person smell them and see what they bring forth in terms of memory. See if you can come up with a specific emotionally

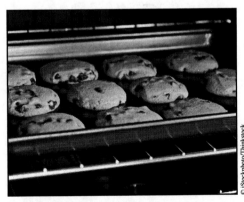

© iStockphoto/Thinkstock.

**Distinctive smells can bring up memories, allowing you to revisit the feelings you experienced then.**

charged incident associated with a scent. Use that memory to re-create and express the feelings aroused at that time.

Here is a third exercise of your emotional memory. Look at a picture of yourself taken when you were half your current age. Then write a letter from the perspective of you at that time to you now. Write all your concerns about school, career, whether you're going to get married, your friends, and so on. When you're finished, respond with a letter to that earlier you in which you relate how all of the things you were so concerned about resolved themselves and you now have other issues in your life. This exercise, if done in the spirit of playfulness, can unite the emotions of earlier years with current emotions—an integrative process.

The goal of all these exercises is to relive not only the memory of your experiences but also the emotions accompanying those experiences. Create memory exercises of your own, remembering to remain alert to current sensations and link them with similar sensations in the past and the emotions they evoked. If the exercises are successful, you will recover memories of experiences you haven't thought about in years. ∎

## Suggested Reading

LeDoux, *The Emotional Brain.*

McGaugh, *Memory and Emotion.*

## Questions to Consider

1. How does emotional memory differ from other types of memory we have studied in this course?

2. Why is it important to reestablish contact with our emotional memory?

# Enlisting Your Emotional Memory
## Lecture 9—Transcript

Welcome back. During the past 3 lectures we have talked about memory, working memory, and memory techniques. Today we are going to talk about an aspect of memory that we do not usually consider when we think about memory, mainly emotional memory. Despite its importance, most of us have lost touch with how we experienced the world in the past. Let me give you an example. I recently went to a high school class reunion—I'll leave it to you to guess what year it might be. I noticed that some of the people I recognized and some of the people I didn't, some of my good friends I recognized more quickly. We began to reminisce and talk about football games, dances, things like this. We remembered all the incidents and events but the memories of the emotions that accompanied them were not present, not as clear. Or if you could bring them up at all, you had vague memories.

You can experience the same thing by taking out your own high school graduation pictures and looking at them very carefully. Do you remember the feelings that day when you graduated from high school? Or how you felt about the specific classmates in the class picture that you're looking at now? Even those whose faces and names you can remember? But when you think about weren't those feelings critical at that time? You feel disconnected and unable to re-experience your thoughts and feelings from that moment. And that's normal there's nothing wrong with that. It's part of what we're going to talk about today, emotional memory. Isn't that loss of emotional continuity with events of your past really too important to lose? What could be more important than your ability to re-establish contact with your emotional memory?

The acting teacher Constantin Stanislavski defined emotional memory as "that type of memory which makes you relive the sensation you felt when your father died." Stanislavski illustrates emotional memory here by citing an example that almost every one of us can identify with. But obviously not every experience is as emotionally arousing as the death of a father. Other memories are much more mundane and easily forgotten but we pay a price for forgetting too much of our past. If we allow our emotional memories to decline too much we will eventually encounter a stranger staring back at us from our mirror.

Here is an example. I recently met with a patient of mine, an Alzheimer patient, and she had a photo album. We looked at it and went through it. I noticed that she wasn't able to identify people in there. And sad to say she wasn't even able to remember pictures of herself or what they were doing. It was not only that she couldn't remember the events but she had no emotional memory to link with her with her past. No ability to integrate her life experiences. Similar albeit less extreme losses of emotional memory can occur in any of us. Practical consequences flow from such losses, such as generational conflict.

Intergenerational conflict is seen in adults who can't retain an emotional memory or contact with themselves as they were adolescents. That puts them in conflict with adolescent children. This is a reason for conflict between generations, between parents and children, arguments over rules and regulations such as car use, friends, etc. Disagreements about authority and the proper role of government, child rearing practices, the goal of education, all these sorts of things come up as a source of intergeneration conflict, which are based I believe on the fact that the adult cannot really remember what it was like when he was an adolescent.

Emotional contact is harder between generations because the brains of our children are different from our own. Plasticity is the reason. I talked a little bit about that in an earlier lecture when we talked about effective technology. The so called net generation's exposure to media and non-stop digital connectedness is going to result in a different brain structure as a result of the plasticity. As a result they perceive and define reality in ways different from our own. Increasingly frenetic cultures truncate the experience of time too. We discussed that in an earlier lecture, when a person's sense of time and place is altered by technology. Where the now is spread all over the world time wise because of technological changes.

These factors make it all the more important to maintain emotional linkages with our past cultivate our emotional memory. Emotional memory becomes increasingly elusive the further we dig into the past. This loss is gradual;

we talked earlier about graceful degradation meaning it doesn't suddenly go off the map it becomes less clear as time passes. To experience the loss of emotional memory page through some personal pictures starting with something that was taken maybe a few weeks ago on vacation, and something going back a few years. A photo album would be fine, in fact it probably be perfect.

Emotional memory loss can also exist alongside perfectly preserved general memories. We're talking about not about what we talked about in the earlier lectures, working memory and general memory; we're talking about emotional memory. You can have that not working as well as working memory and general memory would be. This results in a developmental blockage. We can no longer communicate with our earlier self the thoughts, feelings, and desires of those earlier times are lost to us. We sort of lose a sense of personal integration.

Constantin Stanislavski also contrasted emotional and general memory via a little story, which he used as a teaching aid: He talked about 2 travelers. He said, 2 travelers were marooned on some rocks by high tide. After their rescue they narrated their impression. One remembered every little thing he did—how, why, and where he went. The other man had no recollection of the place at all. He remembered only the emotions he felt. In succession: delight, apprehension, fear, hope, doubt, and finally panic. The first traveler experienced the incident in purely geographic terms while the other traveler describes his emotions. The first traveler might have suffered from what's called alexithymia, which is called a disorder of emotional experience that we'll talk about more in a few moments.

Stanislavski provides a striking example, also in his book about emotional memory, that we can vividly identify with when first hearing it. Imagine yourself back in 19th-century Russia. It's a winter night and you're inside a nice warm house with a fire. It's a dinner party. In the midst of the dinner party one of the guests turned to the host and says, How's little Boris doing in school? Well, little Boris is the 6-year-old boy who was hit by a carriage about 6 months earlier and been killed. The guest knew this but he had momentarily forgotten it. Now just hearing that story makes you cringe. That is emotional memory?

Why is that story so painful to contemplate? Because it's easy to put oneself into the roles of the main participants: the forgetful guest, the horrified and grief stricken parents. Emotional memory enables us to understand why that scene is so painful for all concerned. We can almost see the stricken faces of the parents the shocked, embarrassed, even angry faces of the other dinner party guests, and then the look of abjection, embarrassment, and regret of the forgetful guest. He said it was something he would never forget and I'm sure it was. We can do this and understand that dinner party situation because our brain processes emotion in the same way as those at the dinner.

Your brain changes whenever you observe in other people the facial expressions typical of the various emotions. Alterations can occur in your brain associated with that emotion. In fact this is a natural, universal language of emotions with people experiencing the emotions felt by another person. A person they either encountered directly or via a picture. Emotions link us with other people this is the basis for empathy. Let me read you a quote from a neurophysiologist from UCLA, Marco Iacoboni. He states, "The way we understand the emotions of others is by simulating in our brain the same activity we have when we experience those emotions."

There's a historical context for this sort of thing of understanding emotions. We want to think about when did scientists first become aware of a link between bodily expression and emotions? The first insight came in the late 19th century. The illustrious Charles Darwin, in a little known book in 1872 called *The Expression of the Emotions in Man and Animals*, observed that each emotion is conveyed by a distinct facial expression and he had photos which showed that across cultures. These emotions that we encounter are usually subtler than the ones seen in these pictures.

More recently we've had the onset of mirror neurons and understanding the mirror neurons in the prefrontal cortex. That came from an experiment in which a monkey was observing another one taking a peanut, eating it, and was noted that the same cells in the monkey observing were the same cells activated in the monkey who was eating the peanut. This is called a perception-action matching system. It's an interesting experiment done in which imagine yourself watching a video of a tea party. And the tea set is put out with cookies and a napkin. Now if you look at that and then a hand comes out and grasps the cup and picks it up. You watch that and then you see another movie in which it looks like the tea party is finished. There's soiled napkin, a little stained tea, the cookies are eaten, and the hand just comes toward the cup but everything is sort of a mess. Well the mirror neuron only responds to the first picture because it's appropriate. Perception action matching system is actually mirroring what the intention is. The intention in the first is to pick up the tea and drink it, the second is just to clean up which is very different. We have this mirroring system; if I'm drinking this tea as you're watching me you'll have activation of the neurons in the sensory part of your brain that will match what's happening to me while I'm drinking the tea. That doesn't mean you can taste my tea but gives you an idea of how we are linked together with these mirror neurons. It's a very profound thought if you think about it, that we are sort of one system. What you do influences me and what I do influences you.

Emotional memory taps into this circuitry experiencing not events but feelings. Emotional memory is associated with the right hemisphere processing as briefly mentioned in the lecture on cerebral geography. Patients with right hemisphere injury, or things not working in the right hemisphere, they can't detect emotions in other people's faces or voices. Sarcasm is lost on them. A phrase like "he's a real brain" doesn't come across with any sarcasm. They think they're talking about an intelligent person instead of saying that person may be a little bit of a nitwit. They also may say insensitive things with hemisphere damage in the right. They have a general loss of emotional interpretive and expressive ability. All from this right hemisphere injury or dysfunction.

Social dissimulation difficult for some people with right hemisphere impairment: They'll say something like "You look marvelous!" when the person looks dreadful is difficult for them to say. There's difficulty with being able to dissimulate emotion. There's great differences however with people in their ability to discern other people's emotions, and conceal their own. Concealment is necessary for harmony we all have a lifetime of practice of concealing our emotions in the interest of preserving harmony. Some people have difficulty even experiencing their emotions. It's called alexithymia. You break the word up into *a-* (without) *lexis-* (word) and *thymos* (feeling) and you find a person who has a real failure in what we would call emotional communication. Emotions are experienced in bodily terms—something happens that would ordinarily be depressive for people they may start complaining of a backache or headache. They also can't fathom other people's emotional responses. Another example of something within the general area of almost normality but there are great variations between people's ability to experience emotion and to express it.

Now emotional memory may not always be conscious. Panic and anxiety attacks under specific and repeatable circumstances may be due to a loss of conscious access to the original experience such experiences of the emotional unconscious occupied psychiatry for many years. Psychotherapy was directed at reconnecting emotions to forgotten or inaccessible memories. Although now we're in the world and age of brain science, we focus on the cognitive unconscious those things that happen outside of awareness, we shouldn't ignore earlier insights that current emotions can be due to emotional experiences in the past that we can no longer remember. Here is an example: Let me introduce you to Lynn, a young woman who worked in the perfume section of a major department store. One evening she took home a sample bottle of a new scent and intended to wear it on her date that evening. She put it on, went out, they went to dinner and the theater. She felt kind of blue and out of sorts. At one point her companion said, You don't seem to be having a good time, is everything ok? She said, Yeah, but I don't really fell like myself. So she went home early. When Lynn got home she was puzzled with the evening's experience. She liked the person she was out with and she liked the dinner, nice play, but she also knew she hadn't been herself. She knew it was something about the perfume but she couldn't put her finger on it. So she started fooling with it. She noticed that lavender was the top note of the perfume. Now a lavender-based perfume had been her grandmother's favorite and Lynn had been raised by her grandmother in the absence of her own mother.

Lynn's experience illustrates the intimate emotionally arousing capacity of smell. Taste is also evocative emotionally. Marcel Proust wrote of this *In Remembrance of Things Past*. This arousing power is based on the direct connections of the olfactory nerves to the amygdala, which is part and a key component of the limbic system. Lynn's pensiveness on her date resulted from the emotional memory aroused by that lavender-based perfume. She felt the stirrings of the emotion of loss but could not immediately identify its cause. Later when she gave full attention to the perfume, the connection with her grandmother became clear to her. At the moment of her insight—and it truly was an insight– she experienced an intense memory of her grandmother along with the emotions of grief and loss that she hadn't experienced in years.

As with Lynn, the emotions that we have experienced in the past are best evoked through one of our senses—the activation of a specific sensory channel. The actress Ellen Burstyn describes the process,

> Let's say I had a situation in a play where I had to experience grief. If I approach it directly, trying to remember some time when I felt grief, the emotion usually retreats. But if I approach it through my senses and I ,say, picture the clothes I was wearing then and see if I can feel the feel of the clothes on my body with my fingertips and then try to remember where in the room I was in and where the light was coming from, and where the window was, see if I can feel the light on my face ... and go through all of the senses ... then as I create all of those various sense memories, the emotional memory will follow.

Other people, compared to Ellen Burstyn, are able to use their memories of the past to invoke emotions. Thus for them emotional memory arises through the act of thinking about past experiences. I'm thinking now of the singer Frank Sinatra who advised aspiring singers to think about and feel what they were singing about. When conveying sadness he thought about a sad event from his life, such as the ending of love relationship. After his breakup with actress Ava Gardner he created in his ballads the pensive longing that immortalized his songs by thinking of Ava Gardner.

In a few moments I'm going to suggest some exercises that may help you to enhance your emotional memory. But first a general observation about the expression and concealment of emotions. I'm going to do it in the form of a question, here it is: If you wanted to decide whether someone is lying to you, would you sooner meet them face-to-face, or would you sooner talk to them on the telephone? Which would you do? Most people would respond they would sooner encounter the person face-to-face. They are convinced they could tell in an instant if the person was lying by doing such things as staring them in the eye. Actually, the telephone is better since emotional leakage is greater in the auditory than the visual sphere. The reason for that is from our earliest years, we've learned to control our facial expressions. It's only actors who can exert similar control over their voices.

I am now going to suggest several sense memory exercises based on the principle that the more vivid the sense memory, the greater the chances of establishing emotional memory. Indeed by trying one of these exercises you can learn much about emotional perception and memory. You may be able to evoke, explore, and even revisit your emotions but approach these exercises in the spirit of play—don't take yourself too seriously and you will have a greater chance of making the exercises work. Here is the first exercise suggested by my daughter Jennifer who is an actress and also a teacher on how to enhance emotional sensitivity. This exercise involves a partner. The two of you sit together on the floor, knees crossed, looking at each other, maybe 2 or 3 feet apart. And you ask the other person to close their eyes and think of an emotion that is very sad. You study their face as they're thinking about this. Then you have them clear their face, think of something neutral. Then have them think of something happy. Observe them carefully, you've previously instructed them not to make any facial movements just think these thoughts. After that's over you become the one that's doing it. You close your eyes; you think this sad thought, the neutral thought, and then the happy thought. Then you open your eyes and repeat it again with the person looking at you. Sad, neutral, happy. Afterwards you compare notes about what you were thinking when you were sad or happy. Then when that person tells you that then you can recheck how you felt about it. Was there anything that you noticed in their face? And then when they had their eyes open, was there anything you saw in their eyes? It's important here not to inhibit facial expression but to remain vulnerable. It's a very unusual opportunity to be able to learn what someone is actual thinking—because she's going to tell you and you're going to tell her—and you're then going to be able to compare that to what you picked up while you were looking at them, or while they were looking at you. The things that she picked up in your facial expression and your eyes that you didn't in hers, and vice versa. The aim is to participate in her experience and her aim is to participate in your experience.

The second exercise involves smell and olfaction, which provides the surest sense for enhancing emotional memory. Proust, as I mentioned earlier, talked about the Madeleine in *The Past Recaptured* in which that evoked strong memories of his childhood. Smell and taste are parts of flavor and they're evocative because of direct connection of olfactory nerve going straight into the brain into the limbic system. Of course that's the explanation as to why perfumes are so evocative as illustrated by the experience of Lynn, who I described a few minutes ago.

This exercise involving scents, you invite some friends to your apartment or home. Each one of the brings something that's a pleasing sensory smell to it, distinctive. Fresh cookies, sandal wood, mowed grass, crayons, doesn't matter what it is. You line these things up and each one of them participates in just smelling it separately and seeing what that brings forth in terms of memory. What does mowed grass make you think of? Does it make you think of summers in upper state New York where you went as a child? Whatever it may be. Crayons—does that make you think of school when you were tiny? Each person describe the memories that each scent evoked along with the emotions that are evoked by smelling these things other things people have brought. The task is to come up with a specific emotionally charged incident associated with a scent. Use that memory to recreate and express the feelings aroused at that time. As I mentioned about the mowed grass, just thinking about mowed grass and being at a summer cottage doesn't do much for you. But when you add that scent of the mowed grass that'll being it forward with an emotional memory.

Here is an experiential exercise based on theater that has potential to provide you with emotional memories 10 years ago. It just so happens that if you draw the muscles on your face back tightly, like this. You can actually reduce your age by about 10 years. For this exercise you do in dimly lit room, quiet, by yourself. You're staring into a mirror like this and you're brain will eventually be able to make some flipping, as we would call flipping back and forth between the way you look 10 years ago and the way you do now. So you can slowly begin to re-experience your emotional responses. There's going to be a playful part of it. As I said you need a quiet, dimly lit room and an openness to your emotional responses. The aim is to experience the body image of 10 years ago let your mind wander and free associate. Think of life circumstances then and now. Enter into the persona of the person in the mirror, you'll encounter random thoughts and images, followed by the emotions.

The process is like looking at one of those ambiguous figures that shift before our eyes from one moment to the next: Like the Salem girl/witch puzzle, where you look at it one way and you see the young woman and then you look at it another way and you see the witch. You can't see them both at the same time. One minute you experience yourself as you are now as you're doing this exercise. The next moment you experience the face starring back at you in the mirror. This is like the ambiguous figure. You can only do this exercise occasionally, by the way the brain eventually catches on and in the absence of novelty and surprise the recovered memories are experienced less vividly. You can do the same thing on a computer if you have access to the computerized photographic technique of morphing. You take 2 photos, one of you 10 years ago and one of you now, laser scan them and by shifting pixels from one photo image to another you can gradually create a transformation. Within seconds and with only a few keystrokes you can detract decades from your current photographic likeness. You are controlling the morphing process and imaginatively re-experiencing yourself.

That's all very interesting but you might say, What's that got to do with science? What's happening in the brain? Let me tell you about an experiment on visual illusions carried out at the University College London. The experiment involved volunteers watching a video of a revolving sphere. They pressed a button and the sphere changed direction. But unknown to them the sphere was not changing direction, it could only be perceived as changing direction. The duration of perceived directional change was recorded as a switch rate. An fMRI was then used to search for activated brain regions. It was found that the superior parietal lobes, up in here the parietal areas, were active. The thicker more interconnected cortex in this region, the faster the switch rate. There are several interpretations of this experiment: That the superior parietal lobe is activating the perceptual illusions. Or superior parietal lobe is conveying an increased ability to note alternative interpretations for the ambiguous sphere. This ability may be genetic or as a result of experience as with architects or others whose work involves mental transformations. I think you can see that it's very similar to that exercise we were doing a moment ago where the brain is seeing itself now and then

10 years ago, flipping back and forth. Whatever the interpretation of the University College London studies may be, they provide some possible explanation for the face exercise described a moment ago.

One more exercise to evoke emotional memory. Look at a picture of yourself taken when you were half your current age. Then write a letter, imagine that you're that person from that you at that time to you at this moment. Write all your concerns about school, career, whether you're going to get married, whether you should get married, about your friends. When you're finished respond with another letter to that earlier you in which you relate how all of the things you were so much concerned about years ago. They finally resolve themselves somehow and that now you have other issues in your life. This exercise if done in the spirit of playfulness, and I want to emphasis again that these are playful exercises, can unite the emotions of earlier years with current emotions, an integrative process. This exercise involves the use of the hand incidentally, because you're writing to yourself so we have further additional input.

The goal of all these exercises is to relive not only the memory of your experiences but the emotions accompanying those experiences. If the exercises are successful you will recover memories for experiences you haven't thought about in years. Create memory exercises of your own, remain alert to current sensations and link them with similar sensations in the past and the emotions evoked by these sensations as with the Ellen Burstyn quote that we went over. Use the power of sensory memory, knowing that the sensations are what stimulate emotional memory. Develop your own methods, and if you do so I suggest you read Konstantin Stanislavsky's *An Actor Prepares*. It is a storehouse of techniques for remembering, resolving, and reliving the emotions that accompanied moments from your past life. He wrote, "Our whole creative experiences are vivid and full in direct proportion to the power, keenness and exactness of our memory."

In the next lecture, we will move from emotional memory to a novel and yet tried and true method for increasing brain performance. Most importantly, this method known as deliberate practice remains entirely under your own control. Thank you.

# Practicing for Peak Performance
## Lecture 10

> Many world-class performers have weighed in on the side of deliberate practice. Marlon Brando, for instance, in a famous interview with Larry King, made the comment [that] with the proper training anyone—literally anyone—could be an actor.

Deliberate practice is the key to improving brain performance and creativity. Neuroscience and psychological research have recently confirmed the effectiveness of this ancient method, which takes advantage of the brain's ability to respond when pushed to the limits. The most important components of deliberate practice are to remain fully aware of what you are doing and to concentrate on those aspects of your performance that you find most difficult.

The goal of deliberate practice is the formation of a flexible memory representation. In one experiment, experienced professional musicians were pitted against good amateur musicians. They were both asked to play under changed conditions. They were asked to play every other note, play using only one hand, or transpose into a different key. Experienced musicians had no problem with that, but good amateurs failed miserably. This experiment illustrates what is meant by encoding and retaining a mental representation: Once it is encoded, it can be manipulated and altered.

In essence, people with extraordinary abilities learn to use their brains differently. For example, chess masters activate their frontal and parietal cortices—the areas involved in long-term memory. Chess amateurs, in contrast, activate their medial temporal lobes—those involved in coding new information. The chess masters are using long-term memory to recognize positions and retrieve their frontal-lobe storage of vast amounts of chess information based on years of practice and learning. Chess amateurs are employing the less effective, case-by-case approach.

Experts develop a long-term working memory. In the lecture on working memory, we defined it as the ability to actively manipulate information. The results of working memory may later be stored in long-term memory depending on our interests and goals. Long-term working memory involves incorporating the accumulated reservoir of information gathered over many years into an instantly accessible form. The degree of expertise depends on how much the person knows and how quickly and easily that information can be retrieved. PET scans confirm increased frontal activity in experts.

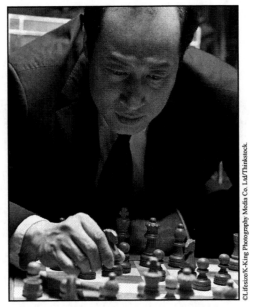

Years of practice allow masters in a field to draw upon long-term memory, making them more adept than amateurs.

Is the ability to form unusually large long-term memories a genetic trait, or is it based on individual effort and persistence? The answer to that question has important implications: If genius is genetic, then most of us are out of luck; but if individual effort is the essential component, then most people are capable of achieving impressive levels of performance. It turns out that deliberate practice is more important than natural talent in determining success.

One piece of evidence comes from a study of musical trainees at the Music Academy of Berlin. It was found that superior students, those who went on to have concert careers, practiced 24 hours a week while good students practiced only 9 hours per week. Similar patterns of long and intensive practice are found among athletes, chess players, mathematicians, and memory virtuosos.

So exceptional performers are not necessarily endowed with superior brains. Rather, the brain, thanks to its plasticity, can be modified by deliberate practice. That approach will enable you to achieve high levels of performance in your area of interest. But to do that you have to be willing to put in a lot of effort. ∎

## Suggested Reading

Restak, *Think Smart.*

## Questions to Consider

1. What distinguishes the approach of an amateur from that of a professional to sports or playing a musical instrument?

2. How many years of deliberate practice does it take to achieve mastery in a particular field of endeavor?

# Practicing for Peak Performance
## Lecture 10—Transcript

Wonderful to have you back for this lecture. Today we're going to talk and speak about something very new about enhancing brain function. It is also paradoxically very old. If you lived in ancient Sparta you would have heard references to what I'm going to tell you, although under a different name. If you were in Japan during the time of the Samurai you would have heard about will and determination. This is essentially what we're going to be talking about under the rubric of deliberate practice. The new part is that neuroscience and psychological research confirm the effectiveness of this ancient method.

I'm talking about deliberate practice, the key to improving brain performance and creativity. Deliberate practice is taking advantage of the brain's ability to respond when pushed to the limits. Today we'll talk about 2 components of deliberate practice that are especially important. First is remaining fully aware of what you are doing. It's funny how many of us go through the day and we're not really paying attention to things, not fully aware of our surroundings or even aware of what's going on inside our minds. The second thing is to concentrate on those aspects of your performance that you find most difficult. Let me illustrate what is meant by deliberate practice. Let's talk a little bit by contrasting the practice methods of professional versus amateur golfers. First of all before we contrast them they have some things in common. They love for the game, they have to be in reasonably good health, and they have to have a desire to excel. The difference involves how each defines and works toward achieving excellence in the game.

Let's talk about the amateur golfer. The goal here is pretty much relaxation and enjoyment—a day out, a day off, a weekend, time like that. Now career advancement can result from the ability to play well, but don't play too well. Don't outperform the boss too often. Golf serves as a social outlet essentially for the amateur player, new people to meet, group identification, travel to distant golf courses, all things like that. Now, the professional golfer has a different orientation. That's because he or she is doing it for a living, the stakes are higher. He or she works on improving weaknesses. First of all to improve a weakness you have to recognize it. And then we're faced with what we call ego issues, nobody likes to think that they can't do everything perfectly. The amateur tends to do the same thing over and over, because he's uncomfortable trying something he's not very good at. The professional doesn't pay so much attention to that. He knows that he's not going to do well in certain things so he's going to work on it. He also resists the compulsion to repeat the familiar. All of us like to do things that we've done before; it's sometimes laughingly called the repetition compulsion.

The goal is to achieve higher levels of control over every aspect of performance. To that extend for the professional, practice is never boring, each day is different. He breaks up what looks like a continual performance into little pieces, when he's putting there's a little placement of the feet, there's a little bit of holding the club a certain way. Nothing is taken for granted, weaknesses are acknowledged they're not denied, and they're addressed through intense practice. But deliberate practice is never easy additional improvements require continuously updating and increased challenges to raise performance beyond the current level. Set challenges for yourself. Make sure you can do better each time you take a particular club and work with it. Now mistakes and failures inevitably result, that's just part of the game. This fact must be accepted and it must be specifically addressed. Failing despite full concentration is painful; it requires renewed commitment—those ego issues again. Are you willing to come back and look at the dark night of what you didn't do very well? The key is to practice things you're bad at, the chances of overall improvement in the whole game are better and vastly improved.

Full concentration is limited to about 4–5 hours, which probably should remind you of what we talked about earlier. When we talked about sleep and rest 6 hours was the thing that was so important. So 4-6 hour range, you can't go much over that and be really doing your best. Many novelists instinctively recognize this and work a few hours in morning followed by spending the rest of the day in relaxed preparation for the next day's writing session. They really can't be talked into working on the same project during the same day; they might take a little time off for writing a story or taking time for a travel article they may be writing. But they're not going to stick with the novel because they realize they've reached the point where they can no longer be productive.

There are 2 requirements for deliberate practice: Full awareness of every aspect of performance, and you get to that by breaking it up into small parts. Of course coaching helps, but it can't be overdone. Imagine a coach following you at every step of the way you're out on the golf course every movement you make he or she comments on it. Well I would think that would be pretty inhibiting. Most people thing would feel the same way. They would say, Well let me work a little bit on my own. The solution is coaching that corrects for major defects but gives you plenty of opportunity to develop your own unique style. For instance concert pianist Angela Hewitt captured this and describes it in her own experience. She wrote, " In my recording sessions I find that the improvement comes not in endlessly repeating a piece, but in listening intently to what has been recorded and then thinking about how it can be done better." That's deliberate practice. Concert pianists, such as Hewitt, eventually reach a point where the essence of their performance is etched in their brain.

The goal is avoidance of automated performance. For example, we all started to learn to drive when we were around 16. We had to put all our energies into steering, using the gears, and the clutches, it was quite a challenge. We got better and then we could sort of listen to the radio or talk to people. Then we became quite experienced, a small number of people went on to become professional drivers, maybe it was trucks or cabs or they went into Formula I racing. But in any case they're goal was a little bit different, they had to take this driving experience and fraction it into smaller and smaller pieces and learn each of those through deliberate practice. Of course there's a goal to all of this: Vigilance and the monitoring of each component of the driving experience. This takes time and most of us who are not professional drivers take it only far enough to drive safely and efficiently under most circumstances. I emphasize most circumstances because that can change and performance can decrease and accidents may result. That's what ice and snow associated mishaps are all about. Somebody living most of the time in Florida, moves up to Vermont for a couple of months and may well be involved in some accidents when we have ice and snow because they're not use to that. The goal of deliberate practice is the formation of a flexible memory representation. Here is an example.

The goal of deliberate practice is the formation of a flexible memory representation. The example is in one experiment in which experienced musicians were pitted against less-experienced musicians. They were both asked to reproduce some tempos under changed conditions. They were asked to play every other note or play using only one hand, or transpose into a completely different key. Experienced musicians had no problem with that while the less experienced ones, the ones we would call very good amateurs, had a lot of problems with it and failed fairly miserably. That experiment illustrated what is meant by encoding and retaining a mental representation. Once it is encoded it can be manipulated and altered. Let's say you're a surgeon. You have encoded in your brain a mental representation; you know the operation you're performing that morning. You go in there and you know how to prepare for it, how to get to the particular organ you're operating on, but sometimes in surgery things don't go just as planned—emergencies arise; things have to be done; different things have to be changed. So the actual order of things sometimes has to be drastically changed. If you're able to adjust to that it's because you have a firm mental representation that can be manipulated. You can adjust to these changes and do things differently if you choose to so. You may look at something and say, Well I'm going to operate a little bit differently today because I think there are things about this operation that require me to make these modifications.

That's what the music studies showed as well. The greater amount of solitary music practice accumulated during musical development and training, the higher the levels of attained musical performance. The more evolved the mental representation for instance that is the music can be broken down into little parts and the components rearranged, and the better you can do that the better you are as a musician.

In essence, people with extraordinary abilities learn to use their brains differently. That's what it is. They actually use them different. For example, chess masters activate their frontal and parietal cortices. Those areas are involved in long-term memory. Chess amateurs in contrast activate medial temporal lobes, those involved in coding new information. Chess masters use long-term memory to recognize positions and problems and retrieve the solutions storage in frontal lobes of vast amounts of chess information based on hard work at least 10 years of practice and learning chess literature and playing. Chess amateurs employ the less effective and their strategy is sort of a case-by-case approach. It's also just not a matter of just amount of info but the speed of retrieval that is important occasionally an amateur will beat a professional. I was actually present when Tigran Petrosian, the former chess champion of many years ago, was playing a multi-player game and there was 1 person was able to beat him out of 40 people. I can assure that if this was lightening chess game this person wouldn't have won. In a lightening chess game long-term memory is being put to short-term use. And a world champion would have a tremendous advantage over an amateur.

Experts develop what's called a long-term working memory (LTWM). Remember in the lecture on working memory in which we defined it as the ability to actively manipulate information. The results of working memory may later be stored in long-term memory depending on our interests and goals. For instance we did an exercise where you went and looked at things. You may want to devise a memory test for yourself instead of doing what was on that particular tape. Maybe makes lists of players or statistics of your favorite professional sports team, something like that. What we had done before was presidents, but maybe the presidents is not much of an interest to you so you use sports figures.

Long term working memory involves incorporating the accumulated reservoir of information gathered over many years into an instantly accessible form. In fact that is a good definition of an expert: a person who increases his long-term memory by many years of practice and then incorporates that knowledge into long term working memory. The degree of expertise depends on how much is known and how fast and easily it can be retrieved. As an example let me tell about Juan Manuel Fangio. Juan Manuel Fangio won the Formula 1 world championship 5 times. He was the first to achieve that level of Formula 1 performance. He raced between 1951 and 1958, when he retired because he was getting too dangerous and the cars were too fast— maybe that's why he did so well, he knew just when to step back. There was a reporter who was doing a story on Fangio; he caught up with him in Monte Carlo in a casino. They both spent some time talking and socializing and perhaps even gambling and having a few drinks. After the interview in the casino, Fangio suggested that they could continue it in the car where he could take the reporter home. So they got in the car, a Mercedes, and they were speeding over 100 mph in the twisting roads outside the city Monte Carlo. Suddenly, as they turned a corner and there was a truck blocking the way. The reporter who wrote about this said he thought this was it, there was just no way of stopping. Yet all things Fangio had learned along the years, breaking, using gear shifts, twisting, everything he used brought the car practically up to the truck and stopped it cold. As the result of many years of deliberate practice, Fangio was able to act instinctively his controlled mental processing had been converted into automatic processing as discussed in Lecture 1. Consciousness certainly wasn't involved; he had no time to think it out. He had no sense of effort. He wouldn't be able to tell anyone exactly what he did; his skill couldn't be explained, only shown.

How many years of deliberate practice does it take to achieve mastery in a particular field of endeavor? I wondered about that for a long time. I finally figured out who I needed to ask. I asked professor K. Anders Ericsson, a psychology professor at Florida State University. He has spent his lifetime studying superior performers in the arts, sciences, and sports. I mentioned him incidentally in the memory lecture, remember student S. F. the track and field performer who could recall 80+ digits? Well he was a student of Ericsson. Ericsson told me about a 10 year rule. He stated that you needed 10 years of deliberate practice and experience. They're both required for expert performance to be achieved in any area. He talked about actors, he talked about fluent speakers, he talked about athletes. Of course, we're all experts in certain things like English. We can remember sentences of 20 or more words. Foreign language only a few, random sequential words even less. Based on what I've told you so far and what you've learned so far in this course, what part of the brain would you suspect is most important in deliberate practice? Think about that, what part of the brain? Here's a little hint: Think of drive, sequencing, executive control, and future memory. The answer of course is the frontal lobes. We think of drive, the determination to stick with the training program. Sequencing is getting everything into the proper sequence for later processing. Executive control is monitoring one's responses and managing separate processes. And finally future memory is keeping future goals in mind and building on the past performances and present abilities.

PET scans confirm increased frontal activity in experts. The German math expert and prodigy Rudiger Gramm showed increased frontal activity when tested. He likes to talk about maintaining a library of notepads, and of course we talked earlier the notebook analogy refers to the frontal temporal lobes. This was not seen in people with underdeveloped math skills. Here's another example of a practitioner of deliberate practice: Gustavo Romero. Several years ago I got a letter inviting me to give a speech at the Mozart Festival in La Jolla. I was pleased and happy to go out there. I did a little reading and discovered that this is an area where the world's experts come about Mozart. I called up the director and said, Well, you know I love Mozart but I don't consider myself an expert. He said, No, come on out we just want you to talk about the brain. At that time I had a book out called *Mozart's Brain and the Fighter Pilot*. Unknown to me Gustavo Romero, who was the performer, had gotten that book thinking it was about Mozart. When he found out it wasn't he read it anyway and loved it and wanted to meet me. So unknown to me he was the one who had invited me out there. After the concert and my talk, he stated there was a party tonight in his honor and would I want to come. This was my opportunity to ask a question that I've always wanted to ask of a concern pianist: How much do you practice? He said, Well, I played Carnegie Hall when I was 12 or 13 and I've always practiced 4–6 hours since then. He stored in his frontal lobes are all the compositions of Mozart.

Now here's a key question for you: What is the relationship between Romero's many hours of practice and his willingness to put in those hours? Is the ability to from larger-than-normal long-term memories a genetic trait? Or is it based on individual effort and persistence. There are important implications that arise from the answer to that question. If genius is genetic then most of us are out of luck, but if individual effort is the essential component, then most people would be capable of achieving levels of performance that will distinguish them from the vast majority of people who are unwilling or unable to put in those 10 years of deliberate practice. What's most important is the decision to make the effort and the resolution to keep to the rigorous schedule. Deliberate practice is more important than natural talent in determining success according to Dr. Ericsson.

He is not alone in that opinion; many world class performers have weighed in on the side of deliberate practice. Marlon Brando for instance in a famous interview with Larry King made the comment with the proper training anyone, literally anyone could be an actor. Know Graham Greene, the novelist, was asked to comment on whether anyone could be a novelist. He stated, "One has no talent. I have no talent. It's just a question of working, of being willing to put in the time." Is there evidence for this new and rather unorthodox opinion? A study of musical trainees at the Music Academy of Berlin superior students tends to support it. They studied superior students, these are people who went on to become concert pianists and have future concert careers. They practiced 24 practice hours a week. Good students practiced 9 hours per week. Similar patterns of long and intensive practice are found among athletes, chess players, mathematicians, and memory virtuosos.

Here's another way of looking at the deliberate practice issue. Recall in Lecture 1 we talked about automatic versus controlled processing. Controlled is when we take every little piece and give the proper attention to it. Don't rush; spend time to get it right. And eventually when we do that again and again and again, we get to the point that it does become automatic but you don't start controlled. Deliberate practice involves controlled processing taking precedent over automatic processing. Later it will become a little bit automatic, we talked about the surgeon—after a while you know how to do the surgery but if something goes wrong you have to switch back into controlled processing.

Choosing controlled over automatic processing confers performance benefits. There's a famous study called the marshmallow studies of Walter Mischel. They were done with 4 year olds. Let me describe what they were like. Little boys age 4 were sitting in a waiting room with their mothers. They were told that a professor was going to come in, take them into the back room, and ask them a few questions. Low and behold out came a man in white coat who looked a little stern but he was friendly and gracious. He took the little boy back had him in a room and said, Here's a really lovely marshmallow, that's very, very good. I'm going to give it to you. You can eat it now, or if you can wait a little while you'll get a second one. But if you eat the first one, I won't give you the second one.

So then he left the room and the boy was sitting there torn between eating this marshmallow and waiting for a chance at the second one. If the first one was really good maybe that would be enough and he wouldn't need anymore. But if it was really, really good he'd want a second one. So he's fighting with himself about what he's going to do. Should he take this or should he wait? Well you might not guess it but the average wait until the second marshmallow became irresistible was 3 minutes. Now we're talking about 4 year olds. However, 30% held out for 15 minutes and got that second marshmallow. What did that tell you about their personality? What were they like as adolescents and adults? Well this group scored 200 points higher on the SAT. As adults they had more education, higher socioeconomic status, they're less likely to smoke drink or use drugs; they were healthier, wealthier, and wiser in other words.

The marshmallow studies measured the ability of preschool children to forego immediate gratification in the interest of later receiving a greater delayed reward. This of course, relates to our earlier discussions of the frontal lobe and also future memory. Obviously also both are undeveloped at 4 year of age as I've described it—the frontal lobe is developing into adulthood, even as a young adult there are parts of the frontal lobe that are still developing. Nevertheless, 30% of 4 year olds were able to wait 15 minutes. Although no studies were done to explore the question, I suspect that the 4 year olds who held out the longest would be more likely to take to deliberate practice.

We're talking here once again about the power of the frontal lobes. In foreseeing consequences, and preferring more later to less now. If there is a genetic component to top performance perhaps it concerns the power of the frontal lobes and the influence of the controlled-deliberate system that we've talked about. Some people may just be genetically driven to doing this; it's easier for them to do. That is certainly possible but I think it's probably a mix of genetics and deliberate practice. The truth probably involves some little genetic and some larger temperamental predisposition to controlled brain processing. This facilitates deliberate practice obviously. The better you are at this and the longer you stay at it, the better the results.

Now there is one exception that's probably occurred to you. I've already mentioned him and, in fact, Ericsson and people always bring this up. Mozart, he was certainly too young for 10-year rule. Actually there's a lot of dispute about when he actually began becoming acquainted with music.

It could well have been close to 2 years of age, which would mean it's was 8 years—pretty close to the 10-year rule. In any case, remember there's only been one Mozart. Deliberate practice works in most instances.

The take home message here is research is confirming that exceptional performers are not necessarily endowed with superior brains. Rather, the brain, thanks to its plasticity, which we talked about in an earlier lecture, can be modified by deliberate practice. That approach will enable you to achieve high levels of performance in your area of interest. But to do that you have to be willing to put in the effort required to achieve mastery.

In the next lecture, we'll move from deliberate practice to a discussion of those times when it's best to not force things, not to try, not to put in too much time, but just kind of relax, let go. Let the brain take its own course. Or as I like to say, let the brain be the brain. Thank you.

# Taking Advantage of Technology
## Lecture 11

**Think of technological aids as extensions of the brain. Our species, if you go back in history, started with sharpened stones in prehistory and evolved to handwritten scrolls, then to the printing press, pencils and pens, then to typewriters, and finally computer keyboards. Each aid offered an advance in information management.**

You may have heard that the brain operates like a computer, but in fact that's not true. It might surprise you to know that the lion's share of brain processing takes place unconsciously, as when we're dancing or driving a car. If you are learning a new dance step, the worst thing you can do is become actively aware of your feet and where they are. Don't try to micromanage your brain by giving it too much conscious direction. I'm referring here to the cognitive unconscious, which is the mental processing that takes place outside of conscious awareness.

The cognitive unconscious is the main part of our mental processing. It starts at the level of the neuron and extends upward to the level of everyday behavior. For example, neuronal responses in the primary auditory cortex are tuned to the personal meaning of a sound. The more important the sound, the more attuned the cell becomes. You've had the experience of being at a loud party and hearing someone say your name across the room. You hear it, but your friend does not. They didn't hear it because their brain isn't attuned to the sound of your name. This preferential recognition has been measured: Your brain responds to the ring tone of your cell phone more quickly than to other cell phone rings.

Culture, rather than biology, is now the greatest influence on brain development. Our culture is inseparable from technology and has been so since the development of the microchip, which is the heart of modern technology. We use portable computers to extend the brain's power. Software programs enhance our speed of response, our working memory, our imaging ability, our reasoning, and our ability to calculate and abstract.

In the book *Total Recall*, Gordon Bell, who is the principal researcher at Microsoft Research, tells of the power unleashed by combining digital recording, digital storage, and digital search. He writes, "With the speed of modern computers, it has become possible to index every word and phrase in every document and to search all of them in an instant. Indexing is the mechanism by which associative memory becomes possible." Automated research has limitations, of course. A research program isn't able to notice correlations and connections that come naturally to you. You can also recognize opportunities to change the program midstream and look at things from a different perspective.

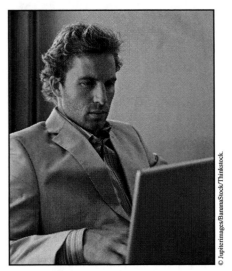

Technology has obvious benefits but can also lead to decreased attention and focus.

There's also a dark side to technology and its influence on the brain. By juggling e-mail, cell phones, laptop computers, and e-books, we're bringing about changes in how our brains operate. We're in the age of distraction, where attention and focus are becoming endangered species. We simply have too many sources of information. The top-down processing by the frontal lobes is interfered with by excessive bottom-up informational processing from the sensory channels. As a result, the deep processing of information is replaced by skimming and surfing.

Nonetheless, the computer has brought about dramatic changes in the way we think. A personal computer brings about a fundamental change in subjective experience: We can link past, present, and future to create personal synthesis and integration. We can revisit earlier thoughts and productions; the you of right now can revisit the you of an earlier time. You can think of it as a form of experiential time travel. ∎

# Video Gaming: Friend or Foe?

Video gaming has burgeoned in recent years: 500 million people around the world now spend more than an hour a day playing video games. The most avid gamers spend 25 hours a week. So what are the positive and negative brain effects of video gaming?

**Pros:**

- Action video games improve peripheral visual attention and enhance eye-hand coordination and reflex responses.

- Video games increase contrast sensitivity, which is important in night driving.

- Games involving teamwork increase collaboration skills.

- Video games can increase some components of IQ. In fact, action video games are more likely to enhance your brain function than the brain gyms that are advertised.

**Cons:**

- There's evidence that video games can be harmful, addictive, and habit forming. Here in the United States, efforts are being made to add video game addiction to the next edition of the *Diagnostic and Statistical Manual*.

- Some gamers experience high intensity immersion, in which they become so absorbed they isolate themselves from everybody else.

- Gamers can experience situated immersion: the illusion of existing within the game. The richness and quality of one's personal life offsets the likelihood of immersion.

So how can you safely enjoy video gaming? First, play no more than 2 to 3 hours per week, and limit your sessions to an hour. Second, avoid games that feature gratuitous violence. Studies have found evidence that violent video games may lead to desensitization to real-life violence. A study of U.S. and Japanese children found that children who play violent games 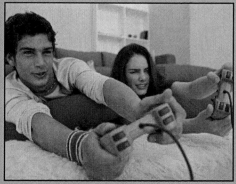 tend to be more aggressive in real life. The challenge is to reap the benefits of action video games while avoiding the potential downsides.

## Suggested Reading

Carr, The Shallows.

Chatfield, *Fun Inc.*

Powers, *Hamlet's BlackBerry.*

Restak, *Mozart's Brain and the Fighter Pilot.*

# Taking Advantage of Technology
## Lecture 11—Transcript

Wonderful to have you back. Today we're going to talk about the brain and technology. You may have heard that the brain operates like a computer, but in fact that's not true. I like to say, just let the brain be the brain, because it's important not to force the brain to work in ways that are counterproductive. Let me give you 2 examples. Those of you who teach, or have taught in the past, recognize that in multiple-choice tests, you have students who are reading the questions over and over, taking fine points and weighing them. Actually for the well-prepared student the best thing is to simply read the question and choose the correct answer.

The second example concerns my daughter. I remember when she was a small child I took her to an eye exam. Those of you who have had your eyes examined, towards the end the doctor's putting a very finely distinguished lens in front of 1 eye: Compare lens A to lens B. When you get to the end of the exam, there's hardly any difference at all. So my daughter asked her if it's lens A or lens B said, Well, let me think it over for a minute. And he said, Well, it's not something you really think over. You just look at it and say whether it is.

So my point is you don't try to micromanage your brain by giving it too much conscious direction. It might surprise you to know that the lion's share of brain processing takes place unconsciously, as in when we're dancing or driving a car. If you learn a new dance step the worst thing you can do is become really actively aware of your feet and where they are. You've got to get into the rhythm of it. Same thing with driving a car.

I'm referring here to the cognitive unconscious, which is the mental processing that takes place outside of conscious awareness. That is the main part of our metnal processing. It starts at the neuron and extends upward to the level of everyday behavior. For example, neuronal responses in the primary auditory cortex are tuned to the personal meaning of the sound. The more important the sound the more attuned the cell becomes. You've had the experience of being at a cocktail party, it's a lot of people and it's noisy. You hear someone say your name across the room and you say to the person you were just talking to, Did you hear someone call my name? They say, No I didn't hear it. They didn't hear it because they're brain isn't attuned to the sound of your name.

This preferential recognition can be measured. Your brain responds to the ring tone of your cell phone within 40 milliseconds of the first ring. That's not true when hearing other cell phone rings. Those examples give you an idea of what I'm talking about when I mention the cognitive unconscious. But I don't want you to think that just because the brains are not mechanistic and that they don't work like computers that we can't take advantage of computers and other technology to enhance our brain function. In fact this lecture we will explore ways to do that.

First of all a very important point: Culture rather than biology is now the greatest influence on brain development. In fact our culture is inseparable from technology and has been so since the development of the microchip, which is the heart of modern technology. We use portable computers to extends the brain's power. Software programs enhance our speed of response, our working memory, our imaging ability, our reasoning, our ability to calculate, and also abstraction. Think of technological aids as extensions of the brain. Our species, if you go back in history, started with sharpened stones in prehistory and evolved to handwritten scrolls, then to the printing press, pencils and pens, then to the typewriters, and finally computer keyboards. Each aid offered an advance in information management.

Let's talk a little bit about the history of information management, because we have an evolution of possible ways to remember something. Back in history people heard something and then they sustained it in their short-term memory then moved it to long-term memory. That's how we have the Homeric epics. Later we started writing things down and dictating notes about them, still later came the typewriter then the laptop. All these methods are what we can think of as one stop sources for writing and editing. Or another way of thinking about it is all are extensions of the brain.

Let's look at the advantages and disadvantages of each. Let's start with written journals. It's amazing how many people I've known that have kept journals. I met a woman of 89 years of age who had kept journals since she was 8 years old. She filled 2 whole bookshelves. Written journals are very personal, they're intimate and familiar. We actually see the brain's production in the form of our own handwriting but we have limited access to written journals over time. This woman couldn't find a particular journal that went back 20 or 30 years and you can understand why. Also as we change our handwriting is sometimes difficult to read. Written documents are difficult to index as well. You're trying to find something, you know you wrote something about this a year or 2 ago and you go through a journal and you can't find the correct one. Synthesis and integration are difficult because you can't link and index.

Now compare that to computer journals. With multigigabyte drives you can cross correlate today's entry with everything you have ever written or in fact ever will write. This is a great improvement over our dependency on books, which aren't always available when we want them. Now I have all of my books on my laptop. Thoughts and images of the past influence what I'm writing now. It's really a form of future memory as we discussed earlier—things in the past influences what you're thinking now, and of course that will influence what you're thinking in the future.

In the book, *Total Recall*, Gordon Bell, who is the principal researcher at Microsoft Research, tells of the power unleashed by combining digital recording, digital storage, and digital search. He writes, "With the speed of modern computers, it has become possible to index every word and phrase in every document and to search all of them in an instant. Indexing is the mechanism by which associative memory becomes possible." And as I mentioned, you don't have any indexing when you're writing something in a handwritten journal.

Advantages of electronic journals don't have to deal with handwriting; you can correlate entries via key words. Key word searches turn up surprising connections many times, that's the advantage of surfing as we call it—you come up with connections that you never really thought of. It's also easy to modify and to add something—you can't do that to a journal that was written 10 years ago and there's no space left.

Automated research, of course, has limitations. There are advantages and disadvantages. These search programs aren't able to find correlations and connections that you would yourself, or that would come naturally to you. You can also change the program mid-stream and see things from a different perspective as mentioned in the lecture on puzzles, word games, and humor Nonetheless the computer has brought about dramatic changes in the way we think. A personal computer brings about a fundamental change in subjective experience we can link past, present, and future to create personal synthesis and integration. We can revisit earlier thoughts and productions; the you of right now can revisit the you of an earlier time. You can think of it as a form of experiential time travel.

The computer has a great influence on brain. It's changing the structure and functioning of the brain as a matter of fact. A mobile electronic device frees us from desks and offices. We can be creative and productive anywhere, even on vacation if we want to we can look up something and tabulate it. We can research using cross references via hyperlinks and hypertext. Let me tell you about a personal example of technology enhancing learning. Remember the paper I mentioned a moment ago about the brain recognizing the ring tone of your own personal cell phone? I wondered about that research and the fact that people select their own ring tones. When you got your cell phone you picked on that you thought reflected your personality and that's your ring tone. So I thought what would happen if somebody were to assign a ring tone? Then have them tested and see if the brain would pick it up in 40 milliseconds. I emailed the author who was in Leipzig, Germany. I said, Let's try to test it next time with an assigned ring tone. Within an hour he got back to me and said, I've already done that and came up with the same finding. My point here is that an informational exchange that could have taken days or weeks sped by in an hour.

Let's talk a little about experiential aspects of technology and how technology is changing what's real. I recently watched on You Tube Pablo Casals playing Suite No. 1 of the Cello Suites of Johann Sebastian Bach. Prior to watching this, my knowledge of Casals depended on historical accounts and his recordings. Watching his performance augmented my understanding and appreciation in a very deep way this immediately led me to watch performances of the Suites by Jacquelyn De Pre. Thanks to this on

You Tube I was able to experientially connect in ways that would have been impossible a few years ago. Technology here provides a form of immortality: I can see, hear, and connect with an artist who died in 1973.

There's also a dark side to technology and its influence on the brain. Technology presents impediments to brain enhancement as well as opportunities. In fact, we are now as a *New York Times* article put it "Hooked on Gadgets, and paying a Mental Price." By juggling e-mail, cell phones, laptop computers, and e-books, we're bringing about changes in how our brains operate. We're in the age of distraction where attention and focus are becoming endangered species. Concentration is decreased and distraction increases. We simply have too many sources of information. Marshall McLuhn referred to it as "information overload." The top-down processing by the frontal lobes is interfered with by excessive bottom up informational processing coming up from the sensory channels. As a result of this the deep processing of information replaced by skimming and surfing. Memory is also interfered with because mental focusing is difficult thanks to scattered attention and distraction. Finally, the technology of the Internet, cell phone, texting, etc. encourage multitasking which we discussed in the lecture on attention.

Multitasking arguments pro and con as you recall, I mentioned in that lecture multitasking is a myth. The brain works sequential not concurrent activities. There's also an interference effects with use of same channel, like when you try to listen to something and try to write something at the same time. Perhaps ok if separate channels but it's not ideal by any means. It's better to deal with everything separately. Mental channels can also interfere with physical channels. Imagining one scene while looking at another, like when you're on a cell phone talking about something at home and your trying to envision it while you're actually suppose to be envisioning what's happening in front of you on the highway. That's because of the bottle neck at the frontal lobes and the cerebral geography that we talked about. Every part of the brain is specialized for something therefore you don't want to overload it.

Let's add here a few additional points about multitasking. Hypertext is a good example and that's a form of multitasking. You see the text and you need to evaluate whether I need to leave the main work that I'm working. And if you do you then need to decide whether or not to click on it. If you decide to click on it, then you have to decide when you're going to return to original text. That's sometimes hard to remember, when the original text you don't remember because you've been on so many hyperlinks.

There are pros and cons of internet reading. A 2007 study shows that shifting from one document to another interferes with understanding. We really do better when we do one thing at a time. The cognitive load, which is the information entering working memory, can be exceeded at such times. That's because of the bottleneck in frontal lobes, which I just mentioned. The internet can function as an interrupter as well, whatever you're doing is suddenly interrupted with its emphasis on speed, reading more, and unfortunately retaining less. These online interruptions can be e-mail, advertisements, pop-ups. Of course we all have curiosity about what we're missing; something's happening and we're missing it. So we check e-mail, check the instant messages, and automatic alerts—which in some cases occur 30 or more times an hour. Thirty or more times an hour, think about that. Overall there's a decrease in efficiency due to switching cost, which increase cognitive load. For multitasking the bottom line is depth, clarity, and cohesion of thought take time—time that you just simply have to find. They also require focused attention. All of these are impaired by the multitasking that internet encourages.

What about videos? What effects do they have? What do they induce in the brain? The video screen has evolved from first television screen, to the computer screens, to videogames screen. There is a shift in brain functioning: from left to the right hemisphere. This explains why critical logical thinking is always better from reading text, from reading paper, than it is from reading from a screen. It's been shown in numerous studies when people are learning some information or trying to learn some information, they do much better when they are reading it from a book or paper then when they are reading it from a television. That's because of the imbalance between the left and right hemispheres. Same thing happens in proofreading. An experienced proofreader would much prefer to read in the final parts a final printed copy instead of doing it all on the monitor.

Of course there are benefits from videos. They can make it possible to re-experience an event through multiple sensory channels. Let me give you an example: I photographed the previous winter's 3 blizzards here in Washington, where blizzards are rare. Nothing like it had occurred since 1899. A few months later, I looked at those pictures on a warm sunny day— same terrain, different world. Technology made that possible. You can do the same thing yourself by looking at pictures and videos you've made and comparing them to where you are now, what things are like at the moment.

The most powerful influence of video however, is video gaming. The emergence and burgeoning of video gaming is comparatively recent: 500 million gamers globally spend more than an hour a day playing games. The hard core gamers spend 25 hours a week. The *World of Warcraft* (WoW) has 10 million subscribers, averaging 12.5 hours a week. Forty percent of Americans are regular players with a 60% of them men and 40% women. The average age is not 16, not 17, not 18 but 35. It's safe to say video gaming is here to stay that's all the more reason that we understand the positive and negative effects that happen with video gaming. Some are obvious of course, if you spend 25 hours a week playing videogames that cuts into relationships. It's also escapism. As one video gamer said, "I could either work in a fast-food chain or be a starship captain." Video games do provide an easy route to prestige and social advancement among one's peers. Success playing *World of Warcraft* brings quicker recognition than a high grade in a semester course. In fact some students turn to video games as an escape from academic difficulties.

What are the effects on the brain? What happens when we're doing videogames? First of all they provide immediate performance feedback. A *Nature* study in 2003 showed that action videogames improve peripheral visual attention. There are also enhanced eye-hand coordination and reflex responses. Also increase contrast sensitivity, which is important in night driving when vision is reduced. Games involving teamwork also increase collaboration skills. There is research on video gaming done primarily by Daphne Bavalier and Shawn Green, her assistant, at the Center for Visual Science University of Rochester. They carried out an interesting experiment in which they compared students who did and did not play videogames. They had some problems finding students who didn't play at least some video games. But they kept searching and eventually had a control group. They compared them to the action video gamers. This is the experiment:

Everybody stared at the screen and a random target was flashed in one of 24 possible sites followed by a flooding of the screen with a clutter of objects. Each was asked where had the original target appeared on the screen? Regular video game players were 80% accurate. They could remember and go back through all the chaos that occurred briefly and remember that first flash. Non-players were only 30 % accurate. The attentional blink was also reduced. The attentional blink refers to the time required to detect a second target during a rapid fire target sequence—flashing white flashes at you and suddenly you recognize one and you'll miss the next one or the one after that due to attentional blink.

Subitizing is also improved by 50%. Subitizing is what happens when you go into the supermarket and you're leaving you want to check out, you quickly look at all the different lines and decide which one is the shortest. You don't count everybody, you just sort of say that seems to be shorter so I'm going to get in that line. Of course that has nothing to do with how fast you'll get out of the store but it does show that you can subitize and get into the line that has the fewer number of people in it.

Wisely used, videogames can help you notice more, concentrate better, respond quicker, and increase some components of your IQ. The principle benefits are acquiring specific real-world skills. Airline pilots for at least 20 years have been getting in simulators, which essentially are video games. I've been in myself with pilots and they are very challenging. You think you're actually in an airline cockpit but it's simulated. All the surgeons are able to do some of the surgical operations, some of the procedures on a video game. Also musicians can improve; *Guitar Hero* and other programs can do this.

In fact, action video games are more likely to enhance your brain function than the so-called brain gyms that you see advertised. Video games are more likely to keep your mind and emotions engaged than the repetitive so-called mental workouts provided by the commercial brain training programs. So until we have some solid scientific evidence of the cognitive benefits of these commercial programs, it makes more sense to devote your energies to games you enjoy, where you can use what you know about your emotions and your associative memory.

Now I do want to mention some caveats about video games. There's evidence that videogames can harmful, and addictive, and habit forming. There are cases in Korea of players tracking down and attacking others for killing their avatars. As a result, blackout times have been mandated by South Korea's Ministry of Culture, Sports, and Tourism. The Players have to choose from 3 6-hour black out blocks. During these periods the users are locked out. The ministry is also stepping down on the speed of internet connections for late night players, therefore making the games less playable. These measures are the result of a 2005 case of a 28-year-old man who died after 50 straight hours of playing without stopping to eat or drink. There's also a case of parents who allowed their baby to starve to death while raising a virtual child during 12-hour marathon sessions on *Prius Online*, which is the South Korean version of *Second Life*. There have been 9 additional deaths attributed to online addiction. It's getting so serious that China and South Korea have opened internet boot camps complete with military-style training to get people away from these games. In the UK the first technology-dependence clinic opened in London in mid-2010. Here in the US efforts are being made to add video game addiction to the next edition of the Diagnostic and Statistical Manual, known as DSM.

You're probably wondering why are videogames so potentially harmful? There are 2 reasons. There's things called high intensity immersion, in which you become so absorbed you isolate yourself from everybody else—your 12-hour session in your room by yourself. The second is situated immersion, the illusion of literally existing within the game. Intensity, vividness, and the quality of graphics determines tendency for immersion. Also the richness and quality of one's personal life offsets the likelihood of immersion. There's evidence that unemployed and socially isolated likely to overuse. I also mentioned students who aren't doing well, they will often move on to a video game where they can be more immediately successful. A number of adult over users, and we could call them addicts, now exceeds teens that are overusing in some countries such as South Korea. As I mentioned the South Korea case of parents so addicted to an on-line game they played 12 hours or more at a time to the neglect of their child who died of malnutrition.

There are a couple of ways you can limit the risk of immersion. First of all, play no more than 2–3 hours per week and try to keep it to that. Then limit sessions to not more than an hour. Then I have a way of powering down after a session by applying what I call the Henry James test, remember Henry James the 19th- and 20th-century author who was a bit wordy and sometimes a bit difficult to see where he was going, there wasn't a lot of action—you can use him or other wordy authors that cause you to focus and pay attention to what's going on. There's not a lot of emphasis on fast action. This works as test of your power of sustained attention.

Caveat 2: Avoid games which feature gratuitous violence, especially games based on events like Columbine or Virginia Tech. Douglas Gentile, director of the Media research Lab at Iowa State University, has found evidence from MRI that violent video games may lead to desensitization. The rostral anterior cingulate cortex is important for emotional responses and the frequency of this is less active during a violent game compared to players who don't usually play violent videogames. The ones who are playing the game frequently, they have less action. In other words, those players who are not used to seeing violent images show a strong emotional reaction to those images. This emotional reaction is missing in players of violent videogames. This research suggests that habitual players of violent video games become desensitized to violence in the video games and perhaps even in real life. A study of over 1500 children drawn from the US and Japan found that children who play violent games tend to be more aggressive in real life. We learn what we see and we learn from what we practice.

The challenge is to reap the benefits of action video games while avoiding the potential downsides. That's not as easily done as it appears. I was curious a year or so ago so I spent several months studying the profiles and reading and watching interviews of game designers. Many of them, sad to say, came across to me as a neuropsychiatrist as a bit antisocial, a bit addicted, and very much taken up by reveling in violence. That's certainly not true of all video game players.

Now let's emphasize the positives. You get decreased overall reaction times, increased eye-hand coordination, enhanced manual dexterity, improved spatial visualization, you're better able to work in 3-dimensions, you can divide and rapidly switch attention, and you also increase the number of things you can visually attend to at one time. Going forward, our society will get the video games it demands. Let's think positively and emphasize the positive aspects of video gaming. According to researcher Shawn Greene, "Video-game research is opening a fascinating window into the amazing capability of the brain and behavior to be reshaped by experience." We have positive applications of video games. They include games in which you have real-world problems. You make a problem into a game. There are opportunities for advancements in status and rewards, it's called leveling up in the game world and it's getting some prestige in a legitimate way. For example, there's a game called Evoke by serious game designer Jane McGonigal, which involves creative collaborations on solving world problems like water safety and food security. Other real-world games include *Darfur is Dying*, which is managing a refugee camp. Or *World Without Oil*, which is responding to a simulated world oil crisis. There's another one called *Play the News*, in which players take on the role of world leaders facing various crises. There's one called *Fate of the World*, which you have to call the shots over the next 200 years of global warming.

Video games can also be employed to improve mental and physical conditioning as with the *Wii Fitness Program* which simulates various sports such as tennis and boxing. The important thing is to find activities that match your own interests and that you will enjoy practicing.

In the next lecture we'll explore more ways to build up your cognitive reserve. Thank you.

# Building Your Cognitive Reserve
## Lecture 12

> Neuroscientists have recently come up with another surprising finding called super-aging. The brains of some elderly people lack tau-tangle formation or have fewer tangles than are typically found in normal aging. ... This has profound implications for our understanding of the aged brain: Perhaps degenerative changes are not inevitable.

W e've learned a lot in this course about how our brain works and how to care for it. In this final lecture, I want to leave you with some straightforward recommendations for things you can start doing immediately to organize your brain fitness. By challenging your brain to learn new information throughout your life, you build up your cognitive reserve. This works the same way as planning for retirement by building up a monetary reserve: You improve your cognitive capacity in later years by acquiring education and knowledge throughout your life and feeding your curiosity.

The more cognitive reserve you've built up over your lifetime, the less you will be affected by brain disease. People with higher cognitive reserve are better at recruiting alternative nerve-cell networks or increasing the efficiency of existing networks in response to age-related changes. Yaakov Stern of Columbia University has found that greater cognitive reserve is linked with greater activation in the frontal lobes. As you've learned in this course, the frontal lobes are key to our most advanced brain functioning. If not stimulated, the frontal lobes function less well as we age.

We want to be really reasonable in our expectations of increasing our cognitive abilities, so keep 2 caveats in mind. First, it's possible that people who start with higher IQs are drawn to activities that will increase their cognitive reserve. Some people of higher IQ may even get increased satisfaction from cognitive stimulation. Second, conditions such as Alzheimer's disease are indeed diseases and in some cases are inherited. But it's better for us to assume we are part of the majority who will benefit from building up our cognitive reserve.

So, what should you do right now? Start with things that you are attracted to do and do well at—but also work on things that don't come so easily. Try things that you usually don't do. If you're a lawyer, get interested in math or physics; if you're already a mathematician, get into literature or history. Whatever you do, the goal is to build the brain you want to live with for the rest of your life.

In choosing projects to build up your cognitive reserve, make sure they are the right ones for you as an individual. If you are a competitive person, poker may be better for you than bridge (where teamwork is important). Practice your reasoning skills, memory training, and speed of processing with puzzles and games. Your quest for cognitive excellence will also be aided by healthy and positive mental states. If you feel depressed or otherwise not right, don't ignore it—try to find out why so you can return to a healthy state.

**Only with practice will you have the best chance of optimizing your brain function.**

Remember to keep things in perspective. Take what the ancients called the long view, linking the past, present, and future. This, of course, involves frontal cortex. Don't waste mental energy on things you can't control; most stressful situations arise when we feel dependent on circumstances we can do little about. Avoid sinking into learned helplessness, which is perceiving yourself as helpless and unable to control stress. The remedy is to focus on decisions that you can make now.

Most of all, beware of golden shackles dilemmas. These are situations in which something is pretty good, you're getting benefits from it, but the situation on the whole is negative. These scenarios can require a painful decision, such as finding a new job or getting a divorce. Keep in mind that the stress of not acting can lead to depression, anxiety, sleep disturbance, memory loss, impaired concentration, and impaired well-being. Don't let momentary feelings govern your behavior. Feelings can affect behavior, but it also works the other way: Behavior can affect feelings. So try doing it until you feel it. If you act enthusiastically, you will begin to actually feel enthusiastic.

A special recommendation I have for you is to develop a magnificent obsession. Successful people often have obsessive character traits; they sometimes use these to their advantage but sometimes use them to fret about things. The antidote is a magnificent obsession. Take up a subject that interests you but is unrelated to your background, education, profession, or life experience. Devote an hour a day to improving your performance in this area of interest.

Please actively practice the exercises that I've suggested during this course. Find ways to tailor them to your own interests so that you'll look forward to practicing them, because only with practice will you have the best chance of optimizing your brain function. ∎

## Optimize Your Brain Fitness with a Healthy Lifestyle

What actions should you take to keep your brain in good condition? Here are some immediate steps you can take.

- Get enough sleep at night, and take naps.

- Eat right and exercise. Both of these are things you can do with friends, which is important because isolation and loneliness can impair brain function.

- Increase your capacity for sustained attention and concentration with attentional exercises. Here, too, you can add a social element, as with playing bridge or chess.

- Increase your finger and hand dexterity: Try Jenga, juggling, model building, video games, playing a musical instrument, or enhancing your penmanship.

- Spend less time watching television.

- Try to maintain a healthy sense of humor. (Humor appreciation has been associated with longevity.)

- Develop an appreciation of different styles of art. It's thought now that different brain areas are activated by different styles of painting.

- Develop an appreciation of different styles of music. Music can elevate your mood and activate regions of the brain involved in emotion, reward, motivation, and arousal. Attend a concert with a friend—or even better, go dancing with friends to combine the benefits of music, socialization, and exercise.

## Suggested Reading

Restak, *Think Smart.*

Stern, "What Is Cognitive Reserve?"

# Building Your Cognitive Reserve
## Lecture 12—Transcript

Welcome back to our final lecture. This is on cognitive reserve. We've learned a lot in this course about how our brain works and how to care for it. In this final lecture I want to leave you with some straightforward recommendations for things you can start doing immediately to optimize your brain fitness. These are things I've learned over a long career as a neurologist, things that I've found that work for me, and what I prescribe for my own patients. The good news, especially for you Teaching Company regulars, is that by challenging your brain to learn new information throughout your life you build up what neuroscientists refer to as cognitive reserve. Research shows that this works the same way as planning for retirement by building up monetary reserve. We improve your cognitive capacity in later years by acquiring education and knowledge throughout our life and feeding your curiosity.

It's an interesting story how we came to appreciate cognitive reserve: About 20 years ago pathologists came upon an unexpected finding in the brains of elderly people. It really surprised them. They found at autopsy the distinguishing hallmarks of Alzheimer's disease in the brains of some people who had shown none of the outward signs of the disease during their lifetime. Up to a quarter of neurons in the cortex were reduced to dense tangled bundles of clusters of degenerating nerve endings enclosing a smudged central core. Alois Alzheimer identified these plaques and tangles as hallmarks of a dementing disease in 1906.

Alzheimer's disease primarily involves memory but, as with Alzheimer's original patient, the symptoms can include many other cognitive processes than memory. Today Alzheimer's disease is the most feared neuropsychiatric illness in the world. We hear about it every day, we read about it in newspapers, we see it in television shows. While memory lapses at any age raise fears of Alzheimer's disease, in most cases such fears are exaggerated. Let me give you an example. It's a weekend and you decide to drive to the mall to do some shopping. You have something particular in mind that you want to get. After parking your car then you go into the store. You're thinking about it and you find what you want. Then you start doing a little more shopping, you go into another store for a little bit more shopping. Maybe you even have lunch there. Then you start to go home and you can't remember where you parked your car. Now it's stress and inattention that are the causes of this inability to remember. It's not memory loss as such because you were focusing on shopping, not parking.

Memory impairment in Alzheimer's disease is much more extreme. You would come out if you had Alzheimer or incipient Alzheimer, and you couldn't recall whether you drove to the mall, whether someone brought you there, whether you came in a cab, whether you came in a car. That's the kind of thing that we're talking about when we're talking about Alzheimer problems with memory.

The brain defect with Alzheimer is the accumulation of debris in the brain. Think of discarded items crammed into an already crowded attic. The tangles look like twisted railroad tracks and are made from tau inside the neurons. The plaques look like gummy globs of material outside the neuron. They consist of a central dark core surrounded by a darker rim. With increasing accumulation of debris, nerve cell communication is disrupted. The nerve cells shrink, they die, and eventually they disappear.

In 1984, not so very long ago, neuroscientists discovered that the plaque is composed of a protein called beta-amyloid. Many researchers today believe that beta-amyloid is the hallmark of Alzheimer's disease. It's also the key to understanding it. So, pathologists began to wonder what was going on when they discovered these Alzheimer changes in the brains of a coterie of deceased elderly who had functioned normally during their last years. Curious, the researchers investigated the lives of these exceptions. They discovered a common trait that is increased levels of education. People with more education were less likely to have been diagnosed with Alzheimer disease during their lifetime. It didn't seem to matter what the subject matter was, they could be studying physics or they could be studying history, it didn't seem to matter. Now what is the explanation for this association? It seems to me that education makes for a more efficient use of brain networks. The more educated you are the more efficiently the brain works. This results in a greater ability to withstand the so far unidentified cause or causes of Alzheimer disease. Cause in truth, we really don't know what's causing it at the moment.

Cognitive reserve is the term coined by neuroscientists for this ability of the brain to function normally despite the inroads of Alzheimer disease. Here's an important point: while education is usually formal, so many years in school, it doesn't have to involve traditional academic subjects. Let me give you an example. About 10 years ago I was in Egypt on a trip with some friends. We had an Egyptologist with us, a small group of people, about 15 people. Over the course of a couple of days it became clear that one of the members of the group, a retired food retailer, knew just about as much about Egypt as the Egyptologist. I asked him later, "Well, how did you learn all this information?" He said, "Well, I first read about Egypt when I was a kid. I kept up my interest, I always read about it, learned about it, attended lectures, attended movies, watched things on television about it." What he had done is to take a magnificent obsession and turn it into a lifetime of self-education. Art Buchwald is another example of this. Art had 2 years of college, yet he had an international reputation as a syndicated columnist and wrote over 50 books.

Think of monetary reserve as a metaphor for cognitive reserve; the greater your monetary reserve the more money you will have available to manage financial reverses. You will have to lose more money before experiencing a financial wipe out. The more cognitive reserve you've built up over your lifetime, the less you will be affected by brain disease. People with higher cognitive reserve are better at recruiting alternative nerve cell networks or increasing the efficiency of existing networks in response to age-related changes.

Cognitive reserve is a lifetime enterprise that starts early. It's not something you are born with but something that you can change all your life and modify throughout your lifespan. Think back to our monetary analogy: It's never too late to start saving, but the earlier you start saving the better. There's a Scottish Mental Health Survey analyzed people born in 1921 who were IQ tested at age 11 and many years later at 80. Although the IQ scores at 11 were strong predictor's of IQ at 80, some respondents significantly increased their IQ. This is an indicator of one of the points I have stressed throughout this course: IQ can be increased. I spoke in more detail about that in Lecture 3. There's also a Swedish Twin Registry, where it was found that people engaged in complex occupations seemed to be protected against Alzheimer disease and other dementias.

Yaakov Stern, of Columbia University, has found that greater cognitive reserve is linked with greater activation in the frontal lobes. After taking this course this should not be a surprise to you since the frontal lobes are key to our most advanced brain functioning. If not stimulated, the frontal lobes function less well as we age. Anything that stimulates the frontal lobes contributes to cognitive reserve.

I want you to keep 2 caveats to keep in mind. We want to be really reasonable here and think about the cognitive abilities. First it's possible that people with higher IQs to start with are drawn to activities that will increase their cognitive reserve. Some people of higher IQ may even get increased satisfaction from cognitive stimulation. The second, Alzheimer's is a disease and I want to emphasis that. Which in some cases comes with some degree of genetic loading, meaning it's strongly inherited. I would suggest Iris Murdoch as a notable example of Alzheimer occurring despite strong cognitive reserve. She not only was one of the greatest novelist of the 20th century, considered one by many literary scholars, but she was also a philosopher. But yet she fell prey to the onslaught of Alzheimer and eventually died of that illness.

Neuroscientists have recently come up with another surprising finding called super-aging. The brains of some elderly people lack tau tangle formation or have fewer tangles than are typically found in normal aging. Changiz Geula of the Super Aging Project of Northwestern University described 9 people older than 80 who performed as well on tests of memory as those of 50 year of age. Now these people were of 80 years of age, keep that in mind. They could recall facts after hearing a story. They could remember for later recall a list of more than a dozen words. As part of the protocol, all agreed to donate their brains for examination after death.

The goal now is to increase the number of participants from the current number of 9 to 50. What's exciting about this is that it's the first study ever with the focus on what is right with the brains of older people. So far we have no explanation for the super-aged it could be environment, life style, or genetics, or perhaps a combination of all 3. It's best to assume it's not all genetics since we have little control over that. We do remain in control of our life style and the environment. Super-aged people fall into 2 groups:

either their brains are almost immune to tangles or they have fewer tangles than most others of the same age. This has profound implications for our understanding of the aged brain perhaps degenerative changes are not inevitable. It's better to assume you are one of the majority who will benefit from building up your cognitive reserve.

So, what should you do right now? First, start with things that you are attracted to do and do well at but also work on things that don't come so easily. Try new and unexpected things, things that you usually don't do. If you're a lawyer get interested in math, physics, geometry; if you're already a mathematician get into literature, read novels, understand history. The goal whatever you do, is to build the brain you want to live with for the rest of your life. Incidentally that's the goal of this course.

To do that you have to recognize your deficiencies, that's difficult for all of us. We all have ego problems to overcome. Nobody wants to admit they are deficient in anything. For example you can ask any group of people, How many of you consider yourself of greater than average intelligence? I can almost guarantee that everyone will put their hand up to indicate yes. Well if that's true then the concept of average intelligence has no meaning.

Let's talk about projects for building up cognitive reserve. First the projects must be individualized. If you are a competitive kind of person, poker may be better for you than bridge where team playing is important. If you retire, retire to something. Your goal is to keep your brain stimulated to increase cognitive reserve. You can increase cognitive reserve by regular engagement in cognitive training. Let me tell you about an example, the research of Michael Marsiske, a lead investigator in a NIH study. He studied subjects ranging in age from 65–90, with an average age of 73. They underwent 10 sessions between 60–75 minutes and he found that was sufficient to boost reasoning skills, memory, and rapid mental processing.

Let's talk a little bit more detail about these 3 areas of improvement found by Marsiske. First, let's talk about reasoning skills. He taught them how to learn to discern patterns in a letter of series of letters. For instance a, c, e, g, i. What's the next letter? It's k, since every other letter has been omitted. These kind of puzzles and games are in a book that I've written recently with Scott

Kim (*The Playful Brain*). The second area that Marsiske was studying was the memory training. He taught his subjects to form visual images, mental associations, and construct narratives. That is similar to the suggestions in the memory lecture—remember the log that was walking along the street and was pick pocketed. Third area is speed of processing, visual searching with divided attention. Subjects were asked to look at a computer and identify objects on the screen at increasingly brief exposure times while dividing their attention on 2 separate tasks. Marsiske's results were very impressive and very dramatic. Just 10 exercises of 60–75 minutes, which is not a lot of time, led to these kinds of improvements: We talked about memory that was improved 75% on memory; reasoning was improved 40%; speed processing was improved 300%. Best of all, remember that these improvements held up over the next 5 years.

Remember these were older adults of average age 73. It's likely that if started earlier the results would have been even better. Formal education is a great asset but adult learning is also effective at a certain point everybody leaves school and becomes an informal learner. What we're doing here in this Teaching Company course is an example of informal self-directed learning. You are taking this course because you want to, no one is standing there forcing you to do it. You are directing your education.

Let's talk now about other concrete steps you can you take. As we proceed remember that the goal is to improve and maintain a general background mental state that is most conducive to achieving top brain performance. Let's start with monitoring your moods, fantasies, and inner talk—the things that you say about yourself and the world. Seek to achieve cognitive excellence aided by healthy and positive mental states. When feeling low, try to discover why. You don't feel the way you should, you feel kind of depressed, try to find why that could be. Try to avoid what I call the buried treasure myth, if you have dig deep down and pull up some psychological reason and say, I must be depressed now because of something that happened 20 years ago. We've sort of moved beyond that psychiatry doesn't really work that way anymore. We think of low moods as a result of things in the environment not events in the past.

Next, keep things in perspective. Take what the ancients called the long view, link the past, present, future. This of course involves frontal cortex. Don't waste mental energy on things you can't control. Most stressful situations arise when we feel dependent on circumstances we can do little about. Avoid sinking into learned helplessness, which is perceiving oneself as helpless and unable to control stress. The remedy is to focus your mental attitude and decisions that you can do now, decisions that you can make. Most of all beware of what I call golden shackles dilemmas that's when something is pretty good, you like it, you're getting benefits from it, but the situation is on the whole negative. On such occasions a painful decision has to be made such as finding a new job or a divorce. Remember the stress of not acting can also lead to depression, anxiety, sleep disturbance, memory loss, impaired concentration, and impaired well being. Don't let momentary feelings govern your behavior. As we know feelings can affect behavior. Ever since we were children we'd say, Well, I didn't feel like doing that. A part of growing up is realizing sometimes you have to do things you don't feel like doing. As Montaigne put it, "Not being able to govern events, I govern myself."

It also works the other way. Behavior can also affect feelings: Do it and you will feel it, we often say. If we feel enthusiastically, act enthusiastically, we will begin to be enthusiastic. There's a quote about that that I'd like to mention. This was taken from William James, who was probably one of the greatest 19th-century psychologists. On the principles of psychology he wrote, "Action seems to follow feeling, but really action and feeling go together, and by regulating the action, which is under the more direct control of the will, we can indirectly regulate the feeling, which is not."

What kind of actions should we take to keep our brains in good condition? Some of it is common sense: get enough sleep, take up the nap habit, eat right and exercise. In terms of eating right and exercising, both of these are things you can do with friends. That's important because isolation and loneliness can impair brain function at any age, so it's important to find ways to engage in activities with other people. Ideally these will be activities you will all enjoy. Company can make even unpleasant activities more bearable, for instance find a companion who will provide you with extra motivation for physical activity.

Next, increase your capacity for sustained attention and concentration. Resist the pressure to multitask but prioritize. Enhance your ability to focus with attentional exercises. And once again when possible, add a social element, as with playing bridge or chess. Work on strengthening your memory. Use but don't depend on digital assistants. Develop a memory system and practice it. Now I had 10 memory pegs, which I talked about in the memory exercise. Things that come to me automatically that I remember in my neighborhood. I have them memorized and then I can take different pieces of information that I want to learn and I can put them on to the 10 memory pegs. You can learn your own memory pegs.

Next, increase your finger and hand dexterity. Jenga, juggling, model building are very helpful. Take up something that requires fingers to be under fine control, like learning to play a musical instrument or trying to enhance your penmanship. Try playing video games, this will increase perceptual acuity and motor responsiveness.

Spend less time watching television. There's a March 2006 study published in the journal *Neurology* compared the cognitive impairment of 5000 people over age 55. It was found that watching TV was associated with a 20% increase of cognitive impairment. We all spend too much of our lives spent with TV. A typical 7year old spends 27 hours per week, by age 70, that means 10 years of life have been spent watching TV. Americans watch 200 billion hours of TV per year, at least they did last year. Good news is there's a huge drop in TV use since cell phones, the internet, and social networks. This has positive implications a computer provides active rather than passive stimulation. As Steve Jobs put it, "You watch television to turn your brain off, and you work on your computer to turn your brain on." So, despite some problems, the Internet is still more stimulating than TV. While TV fosters solitary passive activity, the internet can foster social connections. The purchase of a TV creates one more passive consumer, where as the purchase of a computer or cell phone creates both a consumer and a producer. They both increase the chances of some kind of interaction—networking, e-mail, political action—at least something's happening.

Next, try to maintain a healthy sense of humor. Humor appreciation is associated with longevity in a University of Akron study. The frontal lobes play an active role in the flexible thinking required to get a joke. Also develop an appreciation of art. It's thought now that different brain areas are activated by different styles of painting. In fact, art preferences may be based on brain organization. It's possible to look at a brain images and make a pretty good guess, more than a guess, to be pretty sure whether the viewer is looking at a Dalí or a Picasso.

Similarly, develop an appreciation of different styles of music. Use music to elevate your mood and activate regions of the brain involved in emotion, reward, motivation, and arousal. Neuroscientists at the University of Zurich showed that mood is elevated by listening to 70 seconds of music such as Beethoven's 6th Symphony combined with looking at happiness pictures, such as a smiling man holding a baby. The study showed activation in a distributed emotional network plus parts of the frontal, temporal, and occipital lobes. In a University of Pennsylvania study, mood elevation to music was accompanied by an increase in performance on memory tests. It's speculated that improvement is due to mood-induced increases in attention. So in a way you can think of your iPod as a mood and cognitive enhancer! Listen to music that you find appealing, but experiment with unfamiliar music from time to time. Here again, you can make this a social activity by attending a concert with a friend. Even better go dancing to combine the benefits of music, socialization, and exercise. Dancing leads to improvements in reaction time, posture, balance, attention, nonverbal intelligence, fine motor performance, socialization, and synchronizing movements with others, just think of all these things. Plus you can take lessons in new types of dancing and learn new styles.

A special recommendation is to develop what I call a magnificent obsession. Successful people often have obsessive character traits they use. Sometimes to their advantage but sometimes to worry and fret about things. The antidote is a magnificent obsession. Take up a subject that interests you but is unrelated to your background, education, profession, or life experience. I gave the example earlier of the food retailer who studied Egyptology thorough out his life. Devote an hour a day to improving through practice a specific aspect of your performance in an area of interest.

Many of you may know that I enjoy cooking, for example. I mentioned it in an earlier lecture, I took it up a decade ago and I find it an excellent way of keeping my brain active by using many of the exercises discussed in this course. Cooking provides a practical convenient approach to optimizing brain fitness. The goal is to prepare a meal so that everything is ready on time. It's not always easy to do this because cooking skills tend to decrease with age unless deliberate efforts are made to maintain them. Why is that? Because cooking calls on frontal lobe function which is affected by ageing.

Cooking strengthens and challenges not just the frontal lobes but all of the functions we've been talking about. Let's review some of them and show how that can be. First, improve sensory acuity; get to know herbs and spices. What do they taste like? What do they look like? Where can they be found in the supermarket? Which ones go well with others? Which ones can be substituted for others? And finally, which ones never to put together?

Second, improve sensory memory. Your experience with herbs, spices, and specific foods will enable you to imaginatively create in your mind how a dish will taste simply by reading the recipe. This take time it won't come easily, but with perseverance you can do it.

Third it improves fine motor skills with slicing, dicing, grating, chopping, mincing, julienning separating eggs, measuring. Also the presentation, the aesthetics of the food. How does it look? What are the colors? Fine decorating, as in desserts specifically.

Fourth it improves attention. Direct attention to the recipe with concentrated focus on the directions. Look for terms or procedures you don't understand. Is recipe doable given your current knowledge and skills? Don't try to cook everything. For instance, I don't make pastry. I've given up on pastry I always go out and buy pastry.

Fifth it improves working memory. Balance your time and resources as necessary. If you're going to make a shrimp pasta, the pasta is going to take longer to cook than shrimp so start it first. As you work, focus on how the food will look and how it will taste. And don't forget about one dish while working on another.

Sixth it improves general memory. How did the dish turn out when you cooked it before? What were the problems? I keep a recipe and preparation book, where I try to have the recipe and a picture of what it looked like. I like to see the picture of the food. I enter comments about dish afterwards, what I found easy and what I found hard. I even give myself a grade even—A to C, hopefully nothing lower than C. If it's a new recipe, does it remind you of other things you've cooked before? How did they turn out?

Seventh it improves the frontal lobes, sequencing and anticipating is really great. You have to function as a sous chef, before you get to be the full time chef. You have to have everything ready so it comes together at the proper time. All components are ready to serve, everybody's happy. You also have to make changes and you have to improvise. If you decide to make a salmon dish and salmon isn't available, you have to substitute halibut or striped bass. And know that you can do that, can't do it with just any fish. Try new things but retain insight and humor about your current limitations. When a dish doesn't turn out ask a more experienced cook what he or she thinks went wrong. Formal lessons might be helpful, I've never done that but I'm sure it's helpful, but it's probably not necessary for your goal here to optimize brain function, having some fun with other people, socialize, and also enjoying a good meal.

That's my recipe for maintaining brain health. There are other things one might choose to do hunting, fishing, playing a game or things like that, but please actively practice the exercises that I've suggested during this course. Find ways to tailor them to your own interests, so you'll look forward to practicing them. Because only with practice will you have the best chance of optimizing your brain function. Thank you.

# Bibliography

**General References**

Blakeslee, Sandra, and Matthew Blakeslee. *The Body Has a Mind of Its Own: How Body Maps in Your Brain Help You Do (Almost) Everything Better.* New York: Random House, 2008.

Changeux, Jean-Pierre. *Neuronal Man: The Biology of Mind.* Princeton, NJ: Princeton University Press, 1997.

Crick, Francis. *Astonishing Hypothesis: The Scientific Search for the Soul.* New York: Scribner, 1995.

Damasio, Antonio R. *Descartes' Error: Emotion, Reason, and the Human Brain.* New York: Penguin, 2005.

Edelman, Gerald M. *Bright Air, Brilliant Fire: On the Matter of the Mind.* New York: Basic Books, 1993.

Edelman, Gerald, and Giulio Tononi. *A Universe of Consciousness: How Matter Becomes Imagination.* New York: Basic Books, 2001.

Fields, R. Douglas. *The Other Brain: From Dementia to Schizophrenia, How New Discoveries about the Brain Are Revolutionizing Medicine and Science.* New York: Simon and Schuster, 2009. This insightful book points out that the brain cells are outnumbered by glia cells, whose exact total contribution to brain function are at this point unknown.

Gluck, Mark A., Eduardo Mercado, and Catherine E. Meyers. *Learning and Memory: From Brain to Behavior.* New York: Worth, 2008. This is the best overall introduction to learning and memory. It contains a wealth of references as well as excellent descriptions of the different kinds of memory.

Gordon, Dan, ed. *Cerebrum 2009: Emerging Ideas in Brain Science.* New York: Dana Press, 2009. This book, and the one that follows, contains articles written by scientists as well as science writers, covering a broad range of topics and provides an illuminating guide to the 21st century.

————. *Cerebrum 2010: Emerging Ideas in Brain Science.* New York: Dana Press, 2010.

Gregory, Richard L. *Eye and Brain: The Psychology of Seeing.* Princeton, NJ: Princeton University Press, 1997.

Hebb, Donald O. *The Organization of Behavior: A Neuropsychological Theory.* Mahwah, NJ: Lawrence Erlbaum Associates, 2002.

Heilman, Kenneth M. *Matter of Mind: A Neurologist's View of Brain-Behavior Relationships.* New York: Oxford University Press, 2002.

James, William. *The Principles of Psychology, Volume I and II.* New York: Dover Publications, 1950.

Johnson, Steven. *Mind Wide Open: Your Brain and the Neuroscience of Everyday Life.* New York: Scribner, 2004.

LeDoux, Joseph. *The Emotional Brain: The Mysterious Underpinnings of Emotional Life.* New York: Simon and Schuster, 1998.

————. *Synaptic Self: How Our Brains Become Who We Are.* New York: Penguin Books, 2003.

Livingstone, Margaret. *Vision and Art: The Biology of Seeing.* New York: Harry N. Abrams, 2002.

Mahoney, David, and Richard Restak. *The Longevity Strategy: How to Live to 100 Using the Brain-Body Connection.* New York: John Wiley and Sons, 1999.

**Bibliography**

McEwen, Bruce, and Elizabeth N. Lasley. *The End of Stress As We Know It.* Washington, DC: Joseph Henry Press/Dana Press, 2002.

McGaugh, James. *Memory and Emotion: The Making of Lasting Memories.* New York: Columbia University Press, 2003.

Norden, Jeanette. *Understanding the Brain.* DVD. Chantilly, VA: The Teaching Company, 2007. This is a scholarly but accessible and very illuminating description of the details of brain anatomy, physiology, and other aspects of brain function.

Posner, Michael I., and Marcus E. Raichle. *Images of Mind.* New York: Scientific American Library, 1994.

Purves, Dale. *Neuroscience.* 4th ed. Sunderland, MA: Sinauer Associates, 2008. This is a challenging textbook that covers the fundamentals of neuroscience in great depth.

Purves, Dale, Elizabeth M. Brannon, Roberto Cabeza, Scott A. Huettel, Kevin S. LaBar, Michael L. Platt, and Marty Waldorff. *Principles of Cognitive Neuroscience.* Sunderland, MA: Sinauer Associates, 2008. This book is an excellent introduction to neuroscience and the brain and provides a wealth of information about the brain.

Reid, Cynthia A., ed. *Cerebrum 2008: Emerging Ideas in Brain Science.* New York: Dana Press, 2008. This book, along with the 2 above edited by Dan Gordon, contains articles written by scientists as well as science writers, covering a broad range of topics and provides an illuminating guide to the 21st century.

Restak, Richard. *Mozart's Brain and the Fighter Pilot: Unleashing Your Brain's Potential.* New York: Three Rivers Paperback, 2002.

———. *Mysteries of the Mind.* Washington, DC: National Geographic Books, 2000.

———. *The New Brain: How the Modern Age Is Rewiring Your Mind.* Emmaus, PA: Rodale, 2004.

———. *The Secret Life of the Brain.* Washington, DC: Joseph Henry Press/ Dana Press, 2001.

Schacter, Daniel L. *Searching for Memory: The Brain, the Mind, and the Past.* New York: Basic Books, 1996.

———. *The Seven Sins of Memory: How the Mind Forgets and Remembers.* Boston: Houghtin Mifflin, 2001.

Stuss, Donald T., and Robert T. Knight. *Principles of Frontal Lobe Function.* New York: Oxford University Press, 2002. This text provides both historical and scientific information regarding the frontal lobe. It's well written and easy to understand.

Sweeney, Michael S., and Richard Restak. *Brain: The Complete Mind; How It Develops, How It Works, and How to Keep It Sharp.* Washington, DC: National Geographic Society, 2009.

Wolfe, Jeremy M., Keith R. Kluender, Dennis M. Levi, Linda M. Bartoshuk, Rachel S. Herz, Roberta L. Klatzky, and Susan J. Lederman. *Sensation and Perception.* 2nd ed. Sunderland, MA: Sinauer Associates, 2009. This is an excellent introduction to the specific perceptual processes of the brain and how perception is translated into brain structure and function.

Zeki, Semir. *A Vision of the Brain.* Oxford: Blackwell Scientific, 1993.

**Brain Development**

Bloom, Paul. *Descartes' Baby: How the Science of Child Development Explains What Makes Us Human.* New York: Basic Books, 2005.

Brown, Stuart. *Play: How It Shapes the Brain, Opens the Imagination, and Invigorates the Soul.* New York: Penguin Group, 2009.

Gopnik, Alison, Andrew N. Meltzoff, and Patricia K. Kuhl. *The Scientist in the Crib: Minds, Brains, and How Children Learn.* New York: William Morrow and Company, 1999.

Siegel, Daniel J. *The Developing Mind: How Relationships and the Brain Interact to Shape Who We Are.* New York: Guilford Press, 1999.

## Brain-Related Topics and Memoirs

Bauby, Jean-Dominique. *The Diving Bell and the Butterfly.* New York: Random House, 2008.

Langston, James William, and Jon Palfreman. *The Case of the Frozen Addicts.* New York: Pantheon Books, 1995.

Levitin, Daniel J. *This Is Your Brain on Music: The Science of a Human Obsession.* New York: Dutton, 2006.

Murphy, Nancey C., and Warren S. Brown. *Did My Neurons Make Me Do It? Philosophical and Neurobiological Perspectives on Moral Responsibility and Free Will.* New York: Oxford University Press, 2007.

Newberg, Andrew B., Eugene G. D'Aquili, and Vince Rause. *Why God Won't Go Away: Brain Science and the Biology of Belief.* New York: Random House, 2002.

Sapolsky, Robert M. *A Primate's Memoir: A Neuroscientist's Unconventional Life among the Baboons.* New York: Simon and Schuster, 2002.

Tharp, Twyla, and Mark Reiter. *The Creative Habit: Learn It and Use It For Life.* New York: Simon and Schuster, 2003.

## Care and Feeding of the Brain

Arehart-Treichel, Joan. "Obesity Linked to Changes in Cognitive Patterns." *Psychiatric News* 41 (2006): 25.

Barberger-Gateau, P., C. Raffaitin, L. Letenneur, C. Berr, C. Tzourio, J. F. Dartigues, and A. Alperovitch. "Dietary Patterns and Risk of Dementia: The Three-City Cohort Study." *Neurology* 69 (2007): 1921–1930.

Morris, M. C., D. A. Evans, J. L. Bienias, C. C. Tangney, D. A. Bennett, N. Aggarwal, R. S. Wilson, and P. A. Scherr. "Dietary Intake of Antioxidant Nutrients and the Risk of Incident Alzheimer Disease in a Biracial Community Study." *JAMA* 287 (2002): 3230–3237.

Morris, M. C., D. A. Evans, C. C. Tangney, J. L. Bienias, and R. S. Wilson. "Association of Vegetable and Fruit Consumption with Age-Related Cognitive Change." *Neurology* 67 (2006): 1370–1376.

Phillips, Lisa. "A Mediterranean Diet Is Associated with Living Longer with Alzheimer Disease." *Neurology Today* 7 (2007): 1, 17, 20–21.

Pondrom, Sue. "Caffeine and Fish Oil Found Neuroprotective for Alzheimer Disease." *Neurology Today* 7 (2007): 21–22.

"Six Years of Fast-Food Fats Supersizes Monkeys." *NewScientist*, June 17, 2006.

Stein, Rob. "A Compound in Red Wine Makes Fat Mice Healthy." *The Washington Post*, November 2, 2006.

University of Maryland Medical Center Information Resources: Transfats 101. http://www.umm.edu/features/transfats.htm.

U.S. Food and Drug Adminstration. "Revealing Trans Fats." *FDA Consumer*. September-October 2003. Pub no. FDA04-1329C.

## Cognitive Reserve

Katzman, R., M. Aronson, and P. Fuld. "Development of Dementing Illnesses in an 80-Year-Old Volunteer Cohort." *Annals of Neurology* 25 (1989): 317–324.

Scarmeas, N., and Y. Stern. "Cognitive Reserve: Implications for Diagnosis and Prevention of Alzheimer's Disease." *Current Neurology and Neuroscience Reports* 4 (2004): 374–380.

Solé-Padullés, C., D. Bartres-Faz, C. Junque, P. Vendrell, L. Rami, I. C. Clemente, B Bosch, A. Villar, N. Bargallo, M. A. Jurado, M. Barrios, and J. L. Molinuevo. "Brain Structure and Function Related to Cognitive Reserve Variables in Normal Aging, Mild Cognitive Impairment and Alzheimer's Disease." *Neurobiology of Aging* 30 (2009): 1114–1124.

Stern, Y. "What Is Cognitive Reserve? Theory and Research Application of the Reserve Concept." *Journal of the International Neuropsychological Society* 8 (2002): 448–460.

**Cognitive Neuroscience**

Cacioppo, John T., Gary G. Berntson, Ralph Adolphs, C. Sue Carter, Richard J. Davidson, Martha K. McClintock, Bruce S. McEwen, Michael J. Meaney, Daniel L. Schacter, Esther M. Sternberg, Steve S. Suomi, and Shelley E. Taylor. *Foundations in Social Neuroscience.* Cambridge, MA: MIT Press, 2002. This is a veritable encyclopedia of some of the early works on social neuroscience.

Cacioppo, John T., Penny S. Visser, and Cynthia L. Pickett. *Social Neuroscience: People Thinking about Thinking People.* Cambridge, MA: MIT Press, 2006. This contains now classic papers on social neuroscience and is an excellent introduction to the field.

Gazzaniga, Michael S. The *Social Brain: Discovering the Networks of the Mind.* New York: Basic Books, 1985. This is one of the early attempts to relate brain science to social science.

Hassin, Ran R., James S. Uleman, and John A. Bargh. *The New Unconscious.* New York: Oxford University Press, 2005. This contains important papers by Dr. Bargh, one of the pioneers in social neuroscience.

Restak, Richard. *The Naked Brain: How the Emerging Neurosociety Is Changing How We Live, Work, and Love.* New York: Harmony Books, 2006. This is an early book intended to explain social neuroscience to the nonprofessional audience.

—————. *The New Brain: How the Modern Age Is Rewiring Your Mind.* Emmaus, PA: Rodale, 2003. This is a story of technology and biology converging and influencing the evolution of the brain.

## Consciousness

Baars, Bernard J., and Nicole M. Gage. *Cognition, Brain, and Consciousness: Introduction to Cognitive Neuroscience.* Burlington, MA: Academic Press, 2010.

Edelman, Gerald. *Wider than the Sky: The Phenomenal Gift of Consciousness.* New Haven, CT: Yale University Press, 2005.

Joseph, R. *The Right Brain and the Unconscious: Discovering the Stranger Within.* New York: Basic Books, 2001.

Laureys, Steven, and Giulio Tononi. *The Neurology of Consciousness: Cognitive Neuroscience and Neuropathology.* Burlington, MA: Academic Press, 2009.

LeDoux, Joseph E. *Synaptic Self: How Our Brains Become Who We Are.* New York: Penguin Group, 2003.

Schwartz, Jeffrey M., and Sharon Begley. *The Mind and the Brain: Neuroplasticity and the Power of Mental Force.* New York: HarperCollins, 2003.

## Emotions

Bloom, Floyd, et al. *The DANA Guide to Brain Health.* New York: Simon and Schuster, 2003.

Damasio, Antonio R. *Descartes' Error: Emotion, Reason, and the Human Brain*. New York: Penguin, 2005.

Greenleaf, Robert K. *Creating and Changing Mindsets: Movies of the Mind*. Newfield, ME: Greenleaf and Papanek Publications, 2005.

Griffiths, Paul E. *What Emotions Really Are: The Problem of Psychological Categories*. Chicago: University of Chicago Press, 1997.

Kagan, Jerome. *The Temperamental Thread: How Genes, Culture, Time and Luck Make Us Who We Are*. New York: Dana Press, 2010.

LeDoux, Joseph. *The Emotional Brain: The Mysterious Underpinnings of Emotional Life*. New York: Simon and Schuster, 1998.

Luria, Aleksandr R. *The Man with a Shattered World: The History of a Brain Wound*. Cambridge, MA: Harvard University Press, 1987.

Ramachandran, V. S., and Sandra Blakeslee. *Phantoms in the Brain: Probing the Mysteries of the Human Mind*. New York: Harper Perennial, 1999.

Stein, Kathleen. *The Genius Engine: Where Memory, Reason, Passion, Violence, and Creativity Intersect in the Human Brain*. Hoboken, NJ: John Wiley and Sons, 2007.

**General Cognition: Learning and Memory**

Dehaene, Stanislas. *The Number Sense: How the Mind Creates Mathematics*. New York: Oxford University Press, 1999.

———. *Reading in the Brain: The Science and Evolution of a Human Invention*. New York: Viking, 2009.

Klingberg, Torkel. *The Overflowing Brain: Information Overload and the Limits of Working Memory*. New York: Oxford University Press, 2009.

Nisbett, Richard E. *Intelligence and How to Get It: Why Schools and Cultures Count.* New York: W. W. Norton and Company, 2009.

Restak, Richard. *The Naked Brain: How the Emerging Neurosociety Is Changing How We Live, Work, and Love.* New York: Harmony Books, 2006.

———. *The New Brain: How the Modern Age Is Rewiring Your Mind.* Emmaus, PA: Rodale, 2004.

Schacter, Daniel L. *The Seven Sins of Memory: How the Mind Forgets and Remembers.* New York: Houghton Mifflin Harcourt, 2002.

Tan, Zaldy S. *Age-Proof Your Mind: Detect, Delay, and Prevent Memory Loss—Before It's Too Late.* New York: Warner Wellness, 2006.

Willingham, Daniel T. *Why Don't Students Like School? A Cognitive Scientist Answers Questions about How the Mind Works and What It Means for the Classroom.* San Francisco: Jossey-Bass, 2010.

**Neuroimaging**

Logothetis, N. K. "What We Can Do and What We Cannot Do with fMRI." *Nature* 453 (2008): 869–878.

Poldrack, R. A. "Can Cognitive Processes Be Inferred from Neuroimaging Data?" *Trends in Cognitive Sciences* 10.2 (2006): 59–63.

Poldrack, Russell A. "Neuroimaging: Separating the Promise from the Pipe Dreams." *Cerebrum 2010: Emerging Ideas in Brain Science.* New York: Dana Press, 2010.

Racine, Eric, Ofek Bar-Ilan, and Judy Illes. "fMRI in the Public Eye." *Nature Reviews Neuroscience* 6.2 (2005): 159–164.

## Plasticity

Nelson, Charles A., Charles H. Zeanah, Nathan A. Fox, Peter J. Marshall, Anna T. Smyke, and Donald Guthrie. "Cognitive Recovery in Socially Deprived Young Children: The Bucharest Early Intervention Project." *Science* 318 (2007): 1937–1940.

Restak, Richard. *Mozart's Brain and the Fighter Pilot: Unleashing Your Brain's Potential.* New York: Harmony Books, 2001.

————. *Think Smart: A Neuroscientist's Prescription for Improving Your Brain's Performance.* New York: Riverhead Books, 2009.

## Stress

Sapolsky, Robert M. *Why Zebras Don't Get Ulcers: A Guide to Stress, Stress-Related Diseases and Coping.* New York: W. H. Freeman, 1994. This is one of the early books on stress that still remains timely and relevant.

## Technology

Carr, Nicholas. *The Shallows: What the Internet Is Doing to Our Brains.* New York: W. W. Norton and Company, 2010.

*Carroll, James.* "Silent Reading in Public Life." *Boston Globe, February 12, 2007.*

Connor, Charles E., Howard E. Egeth, and Steven Yantis, "Visual Attention: Bottom-Up versus Top-Down." *Cognitive Biology* 14 (2004): 850–852.

Powers, William. *Hamlet's BlackBerry: A Practical Philosophy for Building a Good Life in the Digital Age.* New York: HarperCollins, 2010.

Rosen, Christine. "People of the Screen." *New Atlantis* 22 (2008): 20–32.

## Video Games

Anderson, C. A. "An Update on the Effects of Playing Violent Video Games." *Journal of Adolescence* 27 (2004): 113–122.

Anderson, C. A., A. Sakamoto, D. A. Gentile, N. Ihori, A. Shibuya, S. Yukawa, M. Naito, and K. Kobayashi. "Longitudinal Effects of Violent Video Games on Aggression in Japan and the United States." *Pediatrics* 122 (2008): 1067–1072.

Chatfield, Tom. *Fun Inc.: Why Play is the 21st Century's Most Serious Business*. London: Virgin Books Limited, 2010.

Gentile, D. A., and J. R. Gentile. "Violent Video Games as Exemplary Teachers: A Conceptual Analysis." *Journal of Youth and Adolescence* 9 (2008): 127–141.

Green, C. S., and D. Bavelier. "Action Video Game Modifies Visual Selective Attention." *Nature* 423 (2003): 534–537.

Jaeggi, S. M., M. Buschkuehl, J. Jonides, and W. J. Perrig. "Improving Fluid Intelligence with Training on Working Memory." *Proceedings of the National Academy of Sciences* 105 (2008): 6829–6833.

Koepp, M. J., R. N. Gunn, A. D. Lawrence, V. J. Cunningham, A Dagher, T. Jones, D. J. Brooks, C. J. Bench, and P. M. Grasby. "Evidence for Striatal Dopamine Release during a Video Game." *Nature* 393 (1998): 266–268.

Li, R., U. Polat, W. Makous, and D. Bavelier. "Enhancing the Contrast Sensitivity Function through Action Video Game Training." *Nature Neuroscience* 12 (2009): 549–555.

Murphy, R. F., and W. R. Penuel. *A Review of Recent Evidence on the Effectiveness of Discrete Educational Software*. Washington, DC: Planning and Evaluation Service, U.S. Department of Education, 2002.

**Bibliography**

Rosser Jr., J. C., P. J. Lynch, L. Cuddihy, D. A. Gentile, J. Klonsky, and R. Merrell. "The Impact of Video Games on Training Surgeons in the 21$^{st}$ Century." *Archives of Surgery* 142 (2007): 181–186.

# Notes